Transposition of the Great Arteries
25 years after
Rashkind Balloon Septostomy

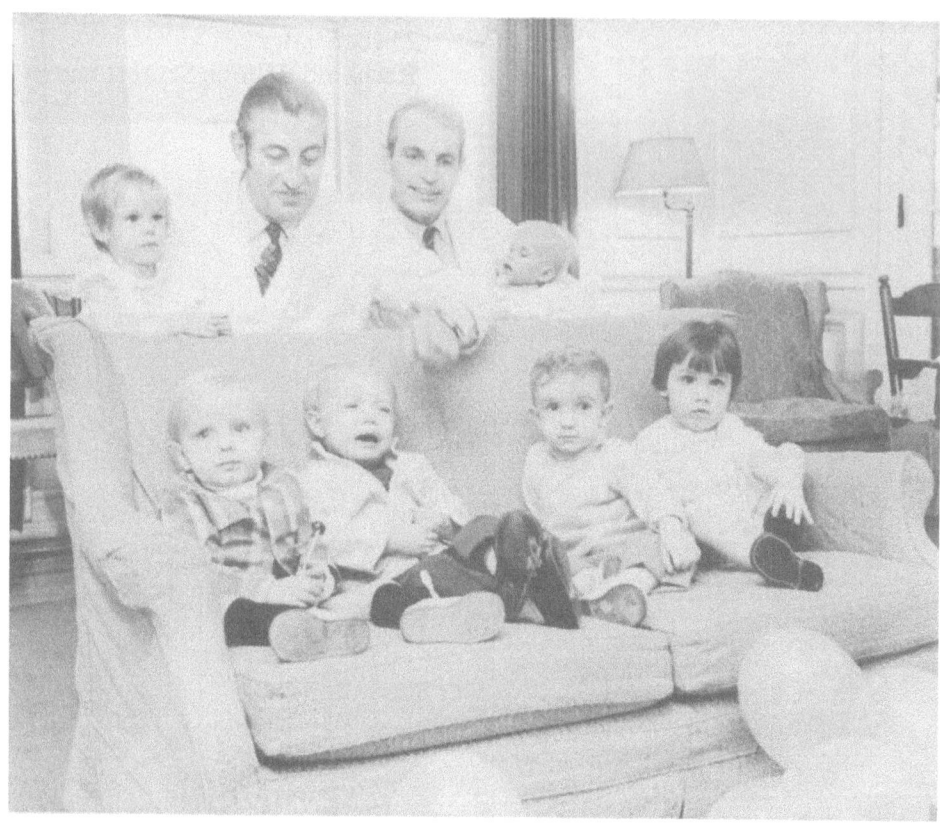

Dr. Rashkind and Dr. Waldhausen, the surgeon for the six first infants who underwent a Rashkind balloon septostomy and, subsequently, a Senning atrial repair for transposition of the great arteries. The dark-haired girl on the right is Melissa Sweitzer, the first patient ever to have undergone a Rashkind balloon septostomy.

M. Vogel, K. Bühlmeyer (Eds.)

Transposition of the Great Arteries 25 years after Rashkind Balloon Septostomy

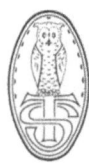 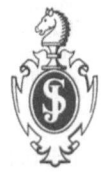

Springer-Verlag Berlin Heidelberg GmbH

The Editors:
PD Dr. M. Vogel
Prof. Dr. K. Bühlmeyer
Kinderklinik
Deutsches Herzzentrum München
Lothstraße 11
8000 München 2

Die Deutsche Bibliothek - CIP-Einheitsaufnahme
Transposition of the great arteries 25 years after Rashkind
balloon septostomy / M. Vogel ; K. Bühlmeyer (ed.). −
Darmstadt ; Steinkopff ; New York : Springer, 1992
ISBN 978-3-7985-0895-8   ISBN 978-3-642-72472-5 (eBook)
DOI 10.1007/978-3-642-72472-5
NE: Vogel, Michael [Hrsg.]

Medical Editorial: Sabine Müller − English Editor: James C. Willis − Production: Heinz J. Schäfer
The use of registered names, trademarks, etc., in this publication does not imply, even in the absence of a specific statement, that such names are exempt from the relevant protective laws and regulations and therefore free for general use.

Printed on acid-free paper

Preface

The international symposium on transposition of the great arteries was held in Munich on May 3–5, 1991. It was organized by the German Heart Center Munich with two aims:

– firstly, to commemorate the 25th anniversary of Dr. Rashkind's publication: "Creation of an atrial septal defect without thoracotomy" (which appeared in 1966 in the Journal of the American Medical Association), and to honor this great pediatric cardiologist, who was one the pioneers of interventional catheterization.
– secondly, to give an overview of current medical knowledge about the pre- and postnatal diagnosis, medical and surgical treatment, and postoperative evaluation of transposition of the great arteries.

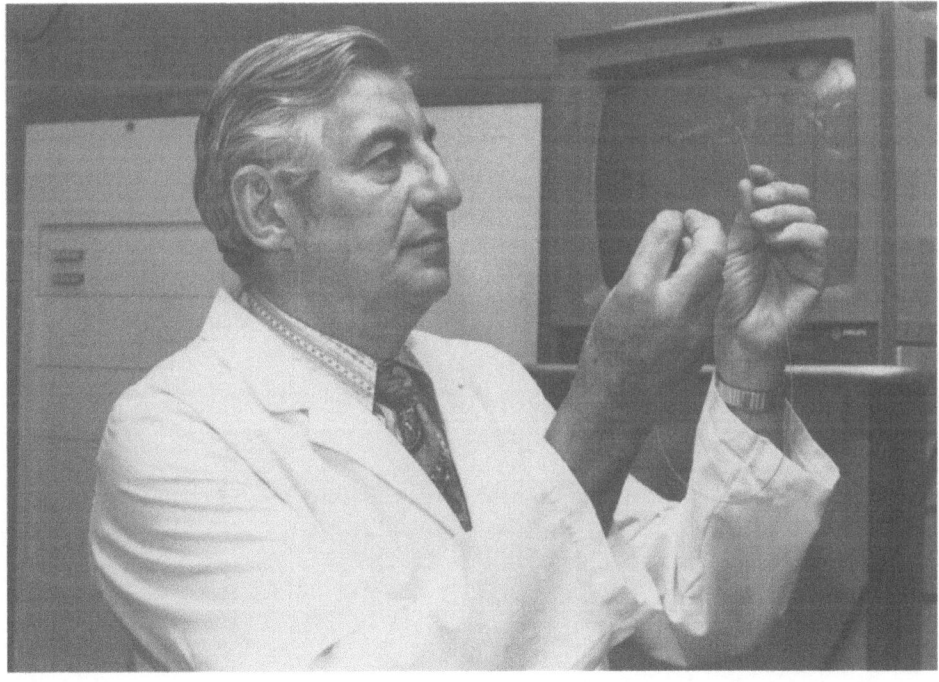

Fig. 1. Dr. Rashkind in his laboratory checking his balloon catheter

This symposium brought together embryologists, morphologists, experts in fetal cardiology, pediatric cardiologists, and pediatric cardiac surgeons from 10 different countries. Thus, we were able to describe the current state-of-the-art of pre- and postnatal management and the surgical treatment of this second most common congenital cyanotic anomaly of the heart.

Dr. Rashkind's approach to create an atrial septal defect in the setting of complete transposition of the great arteries dramatically changed the natural history of this cyanotic heart defect, which carried a 90% neonatal mortality before this effective palliation became available.

His innovative approach literally saved the lives of thousands of cyanotic newborns all over the world. Ingenious new operations introduced by Senning, Mustard and, later, Jatene have made surgical treatment possible and further improved the formerly dismal chances for newborns with this cyanotic congenital heart defect. The current trend to prenatal echocardiographic diagnosis and neonatal surgical repair is an attempt to further reduce the current, already low neonatal mortality. This volume documents the never ending efforts to improve the outlook and prognosis in this heart defect, which requires close cooperation between all those concerned with diagnosis and surgical management of this congenital anomaly.

In closing we would like to thank Drs. Schumacher and Sauer, and the secretaries Mrs. Charaabi and Mrs. Karch, without whose help the organization of this symposium would not have been possible. We also thank Sabine Müller from the publisher Steinkopff Verlag for her kind cooperation in putting together this proceedings volume.

Munich, November 1991   Michael Vogel
                                                              Konrad Bühlmeyer

Contents

Dr. Rashkind: The innovative pediatric cardiologist

Embryology and prenatal diagnosis of transposition of the great arteries

Medical treatment of transposition of the great arteries before surgery

Diagnosis of transposition of the great arteries

Surgical treatment of transposition of the great arteries

Follow up after surgical repair of transposition of the great arteries

Bill Rashkind's contribution to pediatric cardiology

H. R. Wagner
The Children's Hospital of Philadelphia, Philadelphia, USA

I would like to thank Professor Bühlmeyer and his colleagues in Munich for having this meeting dedicated to Dr. William Rashkind. As his longtime friend and colleague, I am greatly honored to share with you a few memories about Bill Rashkind. He was a special friend to many of us around the world, especially here in Europe, where he was a great admirer of the history, culture, and the arts of the Old World.

Bill was born in Patterson, New Jersey, and received his medical degree from the University of Louisville, Kentucky. After graduation he took up the study of cardiovascular physiology, first at the Naval Medical Research Institute at Bethesda, and then in the Department of Physiology at the University of Pennsylvania in Philadelphia. In 1953, he began to concentrate on pediatric cardiology. In 1971, he was appointed Professor of Pediatrics at the School of Medicine, and for many years he served as Chairman of the American Board of Pediatric Cardiology. He lectured by invitation in almost every state of the union and in 35 foreign countries. He earned an international reputation with his balloon catheter, commonly known as the Rashkind procedure.

Personally, I think that his magnificent contribution to pediatric cardiology was that Bill Rashkind used a simple, clinical observation to devise his technique to help children with transposition. He was aware that a large intra-atrial communication was of benefit to infants with transposition. In the early 1960s, he gave a lecture to a group of first-year dental students, covering the entire field of congenital heart disease in one session. In the question and answer period, one of the students applauded the catheters and gadgets Bill had shown and asked why these same instruments could not be used for the treatment of patients rather than for diagnosis alone. Bill took his challenge to "heart". He set himself a new goal: creating an intra-atrial communication with a catheter. First, he used a bent wire, but it failed to tear the tissue of the foramen ovale. Other gadgets were tried: a blade and then a hemostat-like instrument. None of these worked. The break-through idea came on a day when things went poorly. One of Bill's patients developed a clot in the femoral artery after catheterization. The hospital's vascular surgeon came to help and used a Fogarty catheter to extrude the clot from the femoral artery. As Bill watched his colleague, it occurred to him that a rubber balloon blown up in the left atrium and then drawn back across the foramen ovale might indeed solve the problem of creating an intra-atrial communication.

Bill Rashkind's balloon catheter was the beginning of interventional cardiology. During his illustrious career, he also "gadgeteered" a small pump oxygenator. He devised the ductus plug. Later, these handmade creations of metal and foam became larger and more delicate, and he used these to close atrial septal defects. One of the hallmarks of Bill's handiwork was his great determination, extreme per-

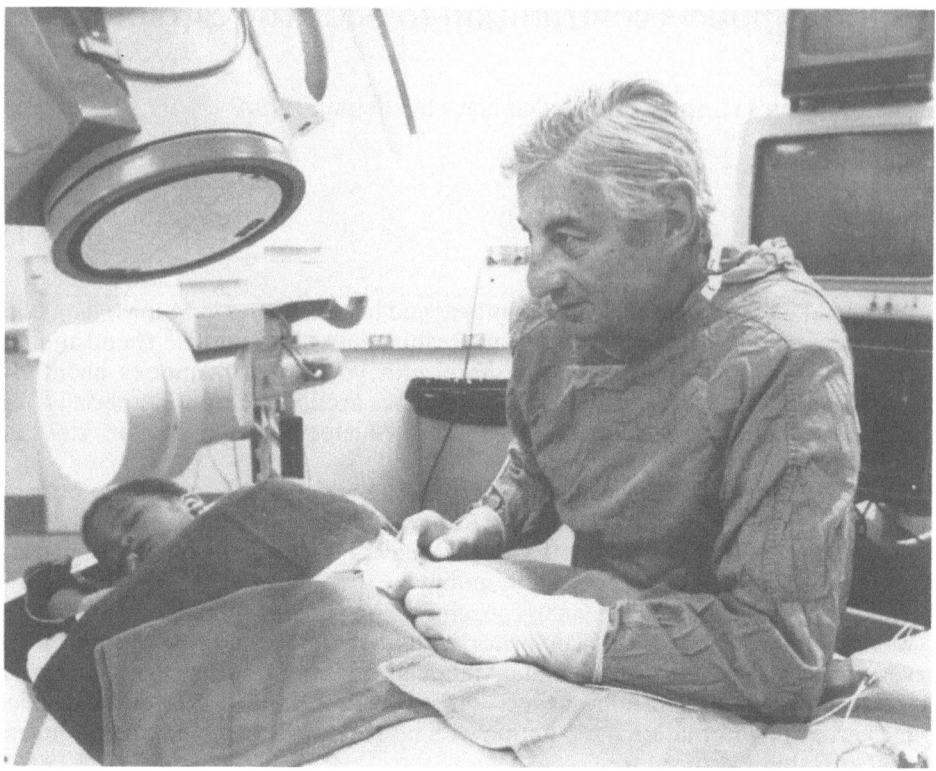

Fig. 1. Dr. Rashkind at work in the cardiac catheterization laboratory

sistence, and tenacity. Bill never gave up. If one of his interventional procedures became tangled after four or six hours, he did not mind going on joyfully for another four. Maybe he yelled "bring me a bigger hammer". About his own malignant disease, he said Henry, "I have big gun disease, but I'm going to fight it". He had a tremendous will to live, but ultimately intense courage to die. Bill taught me as a doctor to fight for every patient, but he also was willing to accept an impossible situation. Bill's professional courage to explore was not unlike Dr. Werner Forsmann, the German Nobel Laureate in Medicine, whom Bill admired religiously. Both pioneers undertook experiments in the spirit of their own conviction, disregarding contemporary dogmatic medical views of risks and feasibility.

Bill was enormously loved by his students for his unpretentious teaching. He gave his best lectures completely unprepared. Before one of his invited lectures, a student dropped Bill's tray full of slides. "Never mind, stuff them back the way you found them", he told the student, and he improvised a one-hour outstanding lecture. Bill's statements were always very simple and, therefore, occasionally less than scientific. He lived after his own Rashkind principle, which he called the KISS principle, which stands for "Keep It Simple, Stupid". One of his historical papers began with the statement, "Children with heart disease are either born with openings too large and others with openings too small". In his only paper on arrhythmia,

2

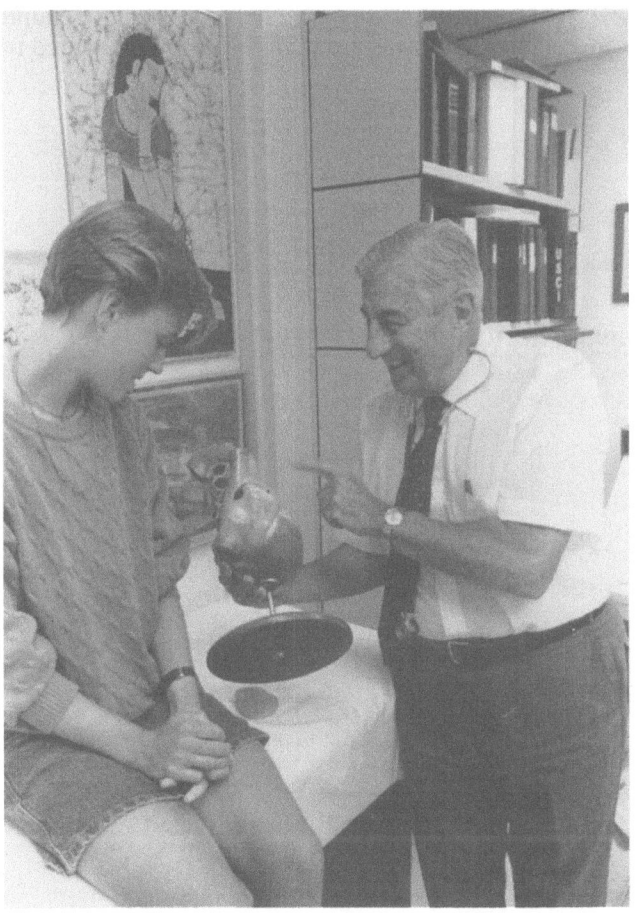

Fig. 2. Dr. Rashkind explains to a mother of a neonate the Rashkind balloon septostomy on a heart model, pointing out the area of the atrial septal defect

he labeled Withering's digoxin as "Shropshire woman's witch brew". On performing a balloon atrial septostomy, he quoted Sylvanus P. Thompson, "what one fool can do, another can". His lectures always started with a historical or pictorial slide: Assyrian tablets, pre-historic cave paintings, a drawing by Leonardo DaVinci, or a Rashkind version of a satirical cartoon from the New Yorker Magazine. If none such was available, it was then a quote by Shakespeare or the Yellow Emperor. His interests in art, culture, and history were sparked by his lovely spouse, Rita Rashkind, herself an art teacher and frequent companion on his world-wide travels.

Many of use were fortunate to know Bill Rashkind personally. We all remember him as a jovial and ever-optimistic friend. His contribution to pediatric cardiology are not only his gadgets, balloons, plugs, and umbrellas, but it is the memory of his unique personality, a true original of the first generation of pediatric cardiologists.

We at The Children's Hospital of Philadelphia are especially proud to have counted him as one of us, and we appreciate that this symposium has been dedicated to a wordlwide friend of us all.

Author's address:
Henry R. Wagner, M.D.
Professor of Pediatrics
University of Pennsylvania
School of Medicine
The Children's Hospital of Philadelphia
34th Street and Civic Center
Boulevard
Philadelphia, Pennsylvania 19104, USA

The impact of Dr. Rashkind on the development of interventional cardiology

M. Vogel, K. Bühlmeyer
Department of Pediatrics, German Heart Center, Munich, FRG

Past, present, and future application of balloon catheters

During the past 8 years the pediatric cardiac catheterization laboratory has changed from a purely diagnostic facility to a therapeutic laboratory, where an increasing number of congenital cardiac abnormalities are treated. This trend originated 25 years ago, when Dr. Rashkind introduced the balloon septostomy technique to palliate critically ill newborns with transposition of the great arteries [26]. Prior to that, Dotter had initiated therapeutic catheterization procedures in adult medicine, when he achieved the first successful transluminal dilatation of peripheral artery obstruction in 1964 [4].

After balloon catheters had proven successful in the palliation of cyanotic heart disease, they were applied to other cardiac lesions. In 1978, Grüntzig introduced percutaneous transluminal coronary artery angioplasty (PTCA), which dramatically changed the approach to adult patients with coronary artery disease [7]. The next major expansion in the application of balloon catheters in 1982 was again achieved by a pediatric cardiologist, when Kan was succesful in treating a valvular pulmonary stenosis with an inflatable balloon catheter [9]. A year later, Lock applied the balloon dilatation technique to treat peripheral pulmonary artery stenosis in pediatric patients [16]. In the same year, Lababidi successfully balloon-dilated a stenotic aortic valve in a child [12]. In 1984, he applied the balloon-dilatation technique to treat native coarctation of the aorta as well [13]. Congenital and rheumatic mitral valve stenosis was treated for the first time by balloon dilatation in the same year, with the intermediate results being better for rheumatic than for congenital mitral stenosis [17]. The technique of balloon dilatation of congenital pulmonary valve stenosis has also been applied to stenosed and calcified bioprosthetic valves in extracardiac conduits with variable success [6, 19]. In the last few years balloon dilation of right-ventricular outflow tract obstruction has included cases with tetralogy of Fallot [23]. This palliation has become popular mainly in Britain, as it may avoid palliation by a surgical shunt, which carries the well known risk of possible distortion of pulmonary artery anatomy. Recently, the technique of balloon dilation has been used in combination with transcutaneous myectomy of the infundibulum in a patient with tetralogy of Fallot [24].

Ballon dilatation of various other congenital heart defects or lesions aquired after surgical treatment of congenital heart defects like tricuspid stenosis [1], subaortic stenosis [35], supravalvar aortic [36] or pulmonic stenosis [33], obstructed total anomalous pulmonary venous return [30], individual pulmonary vein stenosis [5], obstructed venous pathway following Mustard repair of transposition [3], and dilation of stenosed Blalock-Taussig shunts [25] has been attempted with variable success.

The data of the balloon valvuloplasty and angioplasty from 25 North American, 1 European, and 1 Brazilian center were pooled by the VACA (valvuloplasty and angioplasty of congenital anomalies) group and the results up to November 1989 were recently reported [8, 10, 31, 34, 37]. There had been 822 pulmonary and 204 aortic valvuloplasties, and 182 procedures to dilate branch pulmonary artery stenosis, 141 to dilate native coarctation, and 200 angioplasties to treat recoarctation were performed. In the majority of cases pressure gradients across stenosed valves or vessels could be significantly reduced.

Naturally, the history of interventional cardiology is not only full of success, but serious complications have been reported with use of balloon catheters to dilate stenosed valves or vessels. These complications include death during the procedure which occurred in 0.2% in pulmonary [34] and 2.5% in aortic valvuloplasties [31]; 0.7% in angioplasty for native [37] and 2.5% for recurrent coarctation [8], and 2.7% for branch pulmonary stenosis, angioplasty [10]. Complications include perforation of the heart [31], anular tear [34], tricuspid valve tear [34], ventricular fibrillation [31], mitral valve tear [31], pulmonary artery tear [2], cerebrovascular accidents [8], aneurysm formation in the aorta [37], endocarditis [32], and vascular complications with severe femoral artery thrombosis requiring surgical thrombectomy [38]. Most of the complications were age-dependent and occurend more often in neonates and infants than in older children.

For some diseases like valvular pulmonary stenosis, balloon dilatation has become the treatment of choice, whereas it is still investigational in aortic stenosis, especially in the newborn [31] and in native coarctation. Whereas many agree that recoarctation treatment may present an indication for balloon angioplasty, there is still debate in the literature about whether the initial treatment of native coarctation of the aorta should be surgical or by balloon angioplasty [37].

The successful first use of a balloon catheter to palliate a congenital heart defect in a patient was achieved by Dr. Rashkind in 1966. It certainly opened up the field of interventional cardiology and, along with adequate technical modification of the balloons, led to an expansion of the use of balloon catheters.

As the intermediate term effects of treatment of some lesions like peripheral pulmonary artery stenosis and, also, certain forms of coronary artery disease had been disappointing, the use of stents which can be delivered via a catheter system has been introduced [21]. Stents seem to have a benefical effect in some pediatric cases of congenital or aquired peripheral pulmonary artery stenosis [20].

The use of interventional catheters to close congenital heart defects

Balloon catheters have not only been applied to expand stenosed vessels or valves. Detachable balloons have been experimentally used to close arterial-venous fistulae [40]. This application of balloons leads directly to the other field of the rapidly expanding interventional catheter treatment: the closure of congenital or surgically created aortopulmonary shunts via a patent ductus arteriosus or Blalock-Taussig Shunt and atrial or ventricular septal defects. Dr. Rashkind was a pioneer in this field as well. In extensive animal experiments, he began to study the feasibility of closure of heart defects like atrial and ventricular septal defect or patent ductus arteriosus. The first successful closure of a patent ductus in a patient had been achieved in 1967 by Porstman [22]. The device developed by Dr. Rashkind: the

Rashkind ductus occluder (so-called umbrella device), however, is currently the most-widely used occluding mechanism of treat a patent ductus arteriosus [27]. The application of this method has been greatly facilitated by the use of the transvenous approach to deliver the device [28].

Although the nonsurgical closure of atrial septal defects was first attempted in 1976 [11], technical difficulties did not allow a widespread use of this technique. Again, Dr. Rashkind was involved in developing a simple device which could be used for closure of atrial septal defects in children [18, 29]. A collaborative study is currently underway in the USA to evaluate the efficacy and safety of closure of atrial septal defects by use of the Rashkind umbrella device. The same device has recently been used on an experimental basis to treat some forms of ventricular septal defects, but further studies are needed to evaluate the benefits of this method [15].

In summary, Dr. Rashkind's successful use of a balloon catheter to treat atrial septal defects in cyanotic newborns with transposition of the great arteries has opened up a whole new field of interventional pediatric cardiac catheterization. Some of the congenital heart defects like valvular pulmonary stenosis are today rarely treated by surgeons, but rather by pediatric cardiologists. The technique of balloon dilatation of other forms of valvular or subvalvular stenosis and of stenosed vessels remains under investigation. Dr. Rashkind was later very active in inventing practical and easy-to-use catheters to occlude patent ductus arteriosus and atrial septal defects; both techniques are now being subjected to major multicenter trials.

References

1. Bourdillon DV, Hookman LD, Morris SN, Waller BF (1989) Percutaneous balloon valvuloplasty for tricuspid stenosis: hemodynamic and pathological findings. Am Heart J 117:492−494
2. Burrows PE, Benson LN, Moes CAF, Freedom RM (1989) Pulmonary artery tears following balloon valvotomy for pulmonary stenosis. Cardiovasc Intervent Radiol 12:38−42
3. Cooper SG, Sullivan ID, Bull C, Taylor JFN (1989) Balloon dilatation of pulmonary venous pathway obstruction after Mustard repair for transposition of the great arteries. J Am Coll Cardiol 14:194−198
4. Dotter CT, Judkins MP (1964) Transluminal treatment of arteriosclerotic obstruction: description of a new technique and a preliminary report of its application. Circulation 30:654−670
5. Driscoll DJ, Hesslein PS, Mullins CE (1982) Congenital stenosis of individual pulmonary veins: Clinical spectrum and unsuccessful treatment by transvenous balloon dilation. Am J Cardiol 49:1767−1772
6. Ensing GJ, Hagler DJ, Seward JB, Julsrud PR, Mair DD (1989) Caveats of balloon dilation of conduits and conduit valves. J Am Coll Cardiol 14:397−400
7. Grüntzig A, Senning A, Siegenthaler WE (1979) Nonoperative dilation of coronary artery stenosis: percutaneous transluminary coronary angioplasty. N Engl J Med 301:61−68
8. Hellenbrand WE, Allen HD, Golinko RJ, Hagler DJ, Lutin W, Kan J (1990) Balloon angioplasty for aortic recoarcation: Results of the valvuloplasty and angioplasty of congenital anomalies registry. Am J Cardiol 65:793−797
9. Kan JS, White RI, Mitchel SE, Gardner TJ (1982) Percutaneous balloon valvuloplasty: A new method for treatment of congenital pulmonary-valve stenosis. N Engl J Med 307:540−542
10. Kan JS, Marvin WJ, Bass JL, Muster AJ, Murphy J (1990) Balloon angioplasty-branch pulmonary artery stenosis: Results of the valvuloplasty and angioplasty of congenital anomalies registry. Am J Cardiol 65:798−801

11. King TD, Mills NL (1976) Secundum atrial septal defect: nonoperative closure during cardiac catheterization. JAMA 235:2506–2508
12. Lababidi Z, Wu J, Walls JT (1984) Percutaneous balloon aortic valvuloplasty: results in 23 patients. Am J Cardiol 53:193–197
13. Lababidi Z, Daskalopoulos DA, Stoeckle H (1984) Transluminal balloon coarctation angioplasty: Experience with 27 patients. Am J Cardiol 54:1288–1291
14. Ladusans EJ, Murdoch I, Franciosi J (1989) Severe haemolysis after percutaneous closure of a ductus arteriosus (arterial duct). Br Heart J 61:548–550
15. Latson LA, Cheatham JP, Danford DA, Gumbiner CH, Kugler JD, Hofschire PJ (1991) Transcatheter closure of VSD in high-risk pediatric patients. Am J Cardiol 68:426 (abstract)
16. Lock JE, Castaneda-Zuniga WR, Fuhrman BP, Bass JL (1983) Balloon dilatation angioplasty of hypoplastic and stenotic pulmonary arteries. Circulation 67:962–967
17. Lock JE, Khalilullah M, Shrivastava S, Bahl V, Keane JF (1985) Percutaneous catheter commissurotomy in rheumatic mitral stenosis. N Engl J Med 313:1515–1518
18. Lock JE, Rome JJ, Davis R, van Praagh S, Perry SB, van Praagh R, Keane JF (1989) Transcatheter closure of atrial septal defects: experimental studies. Circulation 79:1091–1099
19. Lloyd TR, Marvin jr WJ, Mahoney LT, Lauer RM (1987) Balloon dilation valvuloplasty of bioprosthetic valves in extracardiac conduits. Am Heart J 114:268–274
20. O'Laughlin MP, Perry SB, Lock JE, Mullins CE (1991) Use of endovascular stents in congenital heart disease. Circulation 83:1923–1939
21. Palmaz JC, Richter GM, Noeldge G, Schatz RA, Robinson PD, Gardiner GA jr, Becker GJ, McLear GK, Denny DF jr, Lammer J, Paolini RM, Rees CR, Alvarado R, Heis WW, Root HD, Rogers W (1988) Intraluminal stents in atherosclerotic iliac artery stenosis: preliminary report of a multicenter study. Radiology 168:727–731
22. Porstmann W, Wierny L, Warnke H, Gerstberger G, Romaniuk PA (1971) Catheter closure of patent ductus arteriosus, 62 cases treated without thoracotomy. Radiol Clin North Am 9:203–281
23. Qureshi SA, Kirk CR, Lamb RK, Arnold R, Wilkinson JL (1988) Balloon dilatation of the pulmonary valve in the first year of life in patients with tetralogy of Fallot: a preliminary study. Br Heart J 60:232–235
24. Qureshi SA, Parsons JM, Tynan M (1990) Percutaneous transcatheter myectomy of subvalvar pulmonary stenosis in tetralogy of Fallot: a new palliative technique with an atherectomy catheter. Br Heart J 64:163–165
25. Qureshi SA, Martin RP, Dickinson DF, Hunter S (1989) Balloon dilatation of stenosed Blalock-Taussig shunts. Br Heart J 61:432–434
26. Rashkind WJ, Miller WW (1966) Creation of an atrial septal defect without thoracotomy. JAMA 196:173–174
27. Rashkind WJ, Cuasco CC (1979) Transcatheter closure of patent ductus arteriosus: successful use in a 3.5 kg infant. Pediatr Cardiol 1:63
28. Rashkind WJ, Mullins CE, Hellenbrand WE, Tait MA (1987) Nonsurgical closure of the patent ductus arteriosus: Clinical application of the Rashkind PDA Occluder System. Circulation 74:583–592
29. Rashkind WJ (1983) Transcatheter treatment of congenital heart disease. Circulation 67:711–716
30. Rey C, Marache P, Francart C, Dupuis C (1985) Percutaneous balloon angioplasty in an infant with obstructed total anomalous pulmonary venous return. J Am Coll Cardiol 6:894–896
31. Rocchini AP, Beekman RH, Shachar GB, Benson LN, Schwartz D, Kan JS (1990) Balloon aortic valvuloplasty: Results of the valvuloplasty and angioplasty of congenital anomalies registry. Am J Cardiol 65:784–789
32. Sanyal SK, Wilson N, Twum-Danso K, Abomelha A, Sohel S (1990) Moraxella endocarditis following balloon angioplasty of aortic coarctation. Am Heart J 119:1421–1423
33. Saxena A, Fong LV, Ogilvie BC, Keeton BR (1990) Use of balloon dilatation to treat supravalvar pulmonary stenosis developing after anatomical correction for complete transposition. Br Heart J 64:151–155
34. Stanger P, Cassidy S, Girod DA, Kan JS, Lababidi Z, Shapiro SR (1990) Balloon pulmonary valvuloplasty: Results of the valvuloplasty and angioplasty of congenital anomalies registry. Am J Cardiol 65:775–783

8

35. Suarez de Lezo J, Pan M, Sancho M, Herrea N, Arizon J, Franco M, Concha M, Valles F, Romanos A (1986) Percutaneous transluminal balloon dilatation for discrete subaortic stenosis. Am J Cardiol 58:619−621
36. Tyagi S, Arora R, Kaul UA, Khalilullah M (1989) Precutaneous transluminal balloon dilatation in supravalvular aortic stenosis. Am Heart J 118:1041−1044
37. Tynan M, Finley JP, Fontes V, Hess J, Kan JS (1990) Balloon angioplasty for the treatment of native coarctation: Results of the valvuloplasty and angioplasty of congenital anomalies registry. Am J Cardiol 65:790−792
38. Vogel M, Benson LN, Smallhorn JF, Burrows P, Freedom RM (1989) Balloon valvuloplasty for congenital aortic valve stenosis in infants and children: short-term and intermediate results. Br Heart J 62:148−153
39. Waller BF, Girod DA, Dillon JC (1984) Transverse aortic wall tears in infants after balloon angioplasty for aortic valve stenosis: Relation of aortic wall damage to diameter of inflated angioplasty balloon and aortic lumen in seven necropsy cases. J Am Coll Cardiol 4:1235−1241
40. White RI jr, Ursic TA, Kaufman SL, Barth KH, Kim W, Gross GS (1978) Therapeutic embolization with detachable balloons: factors influencing permanent occlusion. Radiology 126:521−523

Author's address:
PD Dr. M. Vogel
Department of Pediatrics
Deutsches Herzzentrum
Lothstr. 11
W-8000 München 2, FRG

Prenatal pathogenesis of the transposition of great arteries

T. Pexieder, M. Pfizenmaier Rousseil, J. C. Prados-Frutos
Institute of Histology and Embryology, University of Lausanne, Switzerland

Abbreviations used in figures and tables

Ao	Aorta	PAAtr	Pulmonary artery atresia
AoAA	Aortic arches anomalies	PASt/PuSt	Pulmonary artery stenosis
AoInt	Aortic interruption	PGA	Parallel position of great arteries
AoSt	Aortic stenosis	PR	Parietal conotruncal ridge
AoV	Aortic vestibulum	RV	Right ventricle
APs	Aortico-pulmonary septum	sAV	Superior atrioventricular cushion
AS	Aortic sac	SR	Septal conotruncal ridge
ASD	Atrial septal defect	SV	Sinus venosus
AVSD	Atrioventricular septal defect	TAC	Truncus arteriosus communis
CoA	Aortic coarctation	TAPVR	Total anomalous pulmonary
CS	Contruncal septum		venous return
CT	Contruncus	TGA	Transposition of great arteries
DOLV	Double outlet left ventricle	TOF	Tetralogy of Fallot
DORV	Double outlet right ventricle	Tr	Tricuspid orifice or valve
ECD	Atrioventricular cushion defect	V	Undetermined ventricle
FII	Foramen interventriculare		(in A-loop)
	secundum	VSD	Ventricular septal defect
FIII	Foramen interventriculare tertium		
gd	Gestation days		
iAV	Inferior atrioventricular cushion	N.B.:	
LH	Left-heart hypoplasy	SEM micrographs of normal mouse embryonic	
LV	Left ventricle	hearts originate from the work described in	
PA	Pulmonary artery	[61].	

Introduction

Transposition of the great arteries (TGA) is one of the most spectacular cardiovascular anomalies as far as the clinical picture, as well as its treatments are concerned.

The recent epidemiological studies by EUROCAT [41] and by BWIS [14] have shown that TGA represents 7.6 to 8.5% of all children with congenital heart disease seen during their first year of life by pediatric cardiologists (Fig. 1).

The 1986–1987 birth cohorts allow to calculate the prevalence of TGA (Fig. 2). In the EEC countries participating in the Eurocat collaborative study, we recorded 3.54 cases per 10 000 livebirths. Similarly, in BWIS the prevalence was 2.71 per 10 000 livebirths. Interestingly enough, there is very little variation in the incidence of this anomaly over a longer time period and among different epidemiological studies (Fig. 3), the smallest figures being 2.11/10 000, and the largest 3.05/10 000.

Since the first description of a TGA in 1672 by Stenon, its pathogenesis intrigued investigators, who have formulated as many theories as there were reports pub-

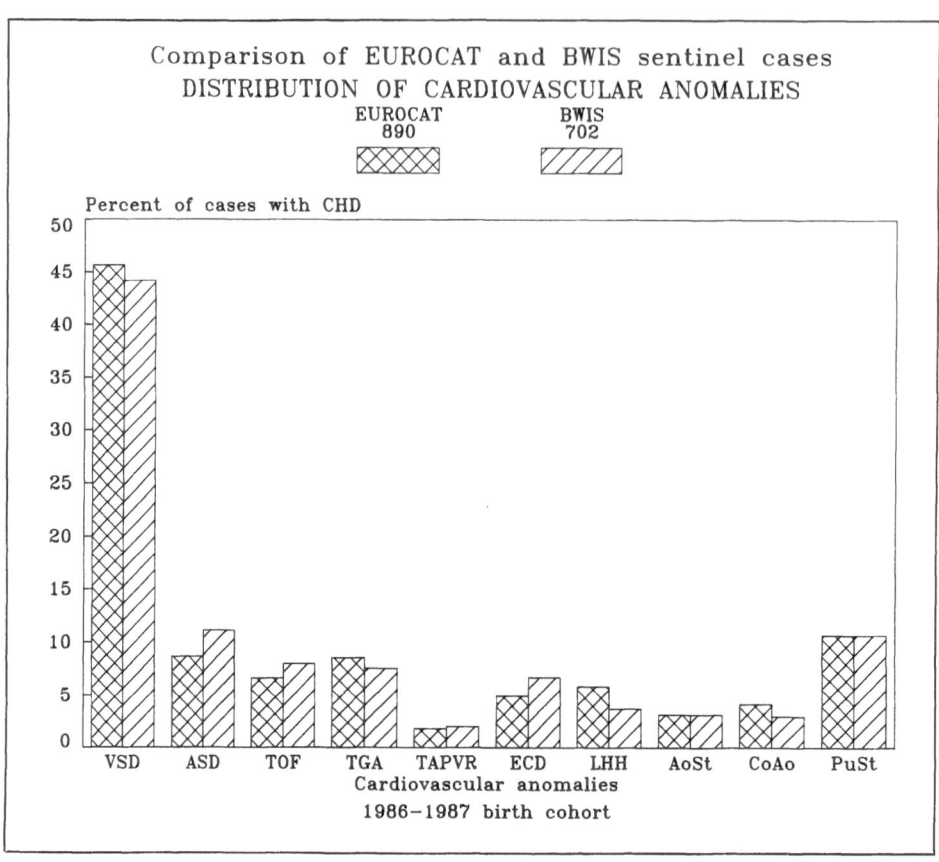

Fig. 1. Comparison of EUROCAT and BWIS sentinel cases, distribution of cardiovascular anomalies

lished on the morphology of this cardiovascular malformation. The most famous of these hypotheses can be systemized either according to the site of primary deviation (Table 1), or according to the postulated involvement of a particular developmental mechanism (Table 2). Considering the site of primary deviation, almost every structure of the developing heart was considered: aortico-pulmonary septum or conotruncus septum, separately or together, or conotruncus septum and ventricular loop. Among the developmental mechanisms considered as being implicated in the pathogenesis of TGA, the following processes were included: rotations and torsions in the conotruncus, absorption in the conotruncus, inversions in the conotruncus, delayed development of the aortico-pulmonary septum, together with a minimal spiralling of conotruncal ridges, or finally looping of the heart tube. Pohanka and Vítek [45] have pertinently characterized the situation by stating that "Most of the embryogenetic theories are purely speculative. Even if they may contain many important descriptive facts, they have to be considered more a conceptual framework for congenital heart disease rather than an explanation of their morphogenesis".

12

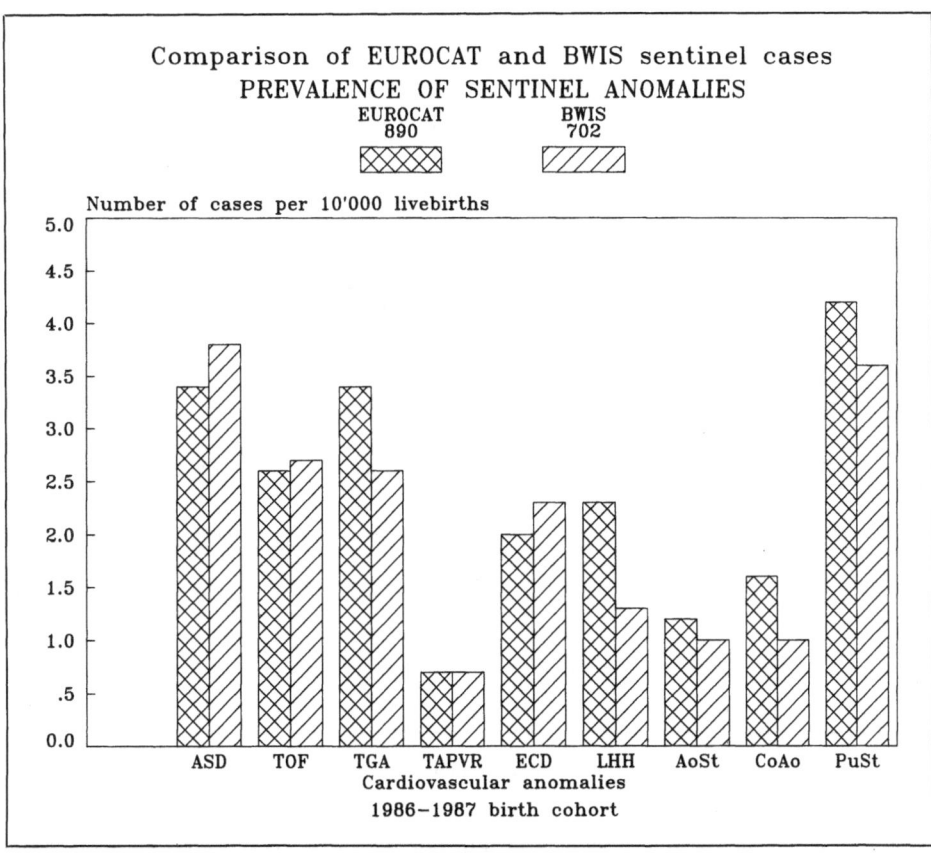

Fig. 2. Comparison of EUROCAT and BWIS sentinel cases, prevalence of sentinel anomalies

One of the reasons why there have been so many theories, hypotheses, and speculations was the absence of an adequate animal model for experimental analysis of the pathogenesis of TGA. As can be seen in Table 3, isolated TGA was only reported by Ueno [56] after rapid neutron irradiation of pregnant rats. TGA as part of a more complete spectrum of cardiovascular anomalies was described after the exposure of pregnant animals to various chemicals, biological factors, as well as physical conditions (Table 3). It is important that the incidence varied from 2.7% with thalidomide [59] to 45.0% with retinoids [19] or 47.5% after hyperbaric hyperoxy [28].

Thus, we decided to develop an animal model of TGA and use it to study, step-by-step, the pathogenesis of this malformation from the time of initial impact of the teratogen until delivery.

INCIDENCE OF SELECTED CARDIOVASCULAR ANOMALIES

per 10,000 livebirths in 6 different congenital heart disease or birth defects monitoring programs

PROGRAM					
New England '69-'77	BWIS '81-'82	Heritage '81-'84	Australia '82-'85	Canada '66-'85	Eurocat '86-'87

ANOMALY					
TGA	2.32	2.11	2.80	2.70	3.05	2.96
TOF	2.14	1.90	1.84	1.00	3.12	2.98
DORV	0.33	0.56	1.45	---	0.85	0.63
TAPRV	0.58	0.83	0.87	0.70	0.75	0.44

Fig. 3. Incidence of selected cardiovascular anomalies

Table 1. Systematics of previously published theories on pathogenesis of transposition of great arteries.

A. According to site of primary deviation	
Aortico-pulmonary septum	Shaner, 1962
	Conte, 1976
	Orts-Llorca et al., 1983
Conotruncus septum	von Rokitansky, 1875
	Robertson, 1913
	Pernkopf, Wirtinger, 1935
	Lev, Saphir, 1945
	van Mierop, Wigglesworth, 1963
	Conte, Arrigioni, 1966
	Bankl, 1971
	Chuaqui, Bersch, 1973
	Anderson et al., 1974
	Chuaqui, 1979
Aortico-pulmonary and conotruncus septum	Shaner, 1962
	Monnie et al., 1966
Conotruncus septum and ventricular loop	Okamoto, 1976
	Sukumar, 1976
	Losekoot et al., 1983

14

Table 2. Systematics of previously published theories on pathogenesis of transposition of great arteries

B. According to developmental mechanism involved

Rotations and torsions in the conotruncus	von Rokitansky, 1875 Robertson, 1913 Pernkopf, Wirtinger, 1935 Shaner, 1962 Bankl, 1972 Chuaqui, Bersch, 1973 Anderson et al., 1974 Chuaqui, 1979
Absorptions in the conotruncus	Lev, Saphir, 1945 Bankl, 1971 Anderson et al., 1974 Sukumar, 1976 Losekoot et al., 1983
Inversions in the conotruncus	van Mierop, Wigglesworth, 1963 Conte, Arrigioni, 1966 Conte, 1976
Delayed development of the aortico-pulmonary septum, minimal spiralling of CT ridges	Monnie et al., 1966
Looping of the heart tube	Okamoto, 1976; Sukumar, 1976 Steding, Seidl, 1984; Losekoot, 1983

Table 3. Experimental production of transposition of great arteries

Isolated				in spectrum			
Neutron irradiation (Day 11–16)	70.0%	Rat	Ueno, 1973	Neutron irradiation (Day 9/13)	10.0%	Rat	Okamoto et al., 1978
				Retinoids		Hamster	Taylor et al. 1978
						Mouse	Davis, Sadler, 1980
					45.0%	Mouse	Irie, Takao, 1990
				Valproic acid	40.0%	Mouse	Sonoda et al., 1991
				Thalidomide		Cat	Khera, Heggtveit, 1974
					2.7%	Rabbit	Vickers, 1960
				Trypan blue	28.1%	Rat	Fox, Goss, 1956
				Antisera		Rat	Barrow, Taylor, 1971
				Hypercapnic hypoxy	1.6%	Rat	Haring, 1966
				Hyperbaric hyperoxy	47.5%	Rat	Miller et al., 1971

Experimental production of transposition of great arteries

We started our experiments by screening 648 rat fetuses, exposed on gestation days 7 to 13 to varying doses (15—300 mg/kg) of retinoic acid, for cardiac and extracardiac anomalies. As can be seen from Table 4, retinoic acid produced a spectrum of anomalies ranging from medium-size ventricular septal defect to parallel position of great arteries and aortic arch anomalies. However, TGA was present only in 1.2% of surviving fetuses when the RA was administered on gestation day 12 [43]. As with the cardiovascular anomalies, each of the extracardiac anomalies (exencephaly, spina bifida, tail, limbs, and face anomalies) peaked according to the day of gestation of RA treatment.

Such a situation, even if interesting from the point of view of experimental teratology, did not correspond to the definition of a good animal model of a cardiac malformation [44]. The low incidence of TGA (Fig. 4) and the presence of a spectrum of lesions (Table 4) were the principal reasons why we switched over to the ICR mouse strain, known for its sensivity to RA and for which, previously, Irie et al. [19] reported rather high frequency of TGA affected fetuses. After some screening experiments, because of the impossibility to duplicate this effect with dosages reported by Irie et al. [19], we chose the RA application by gastric tubing on gestation days 8 and 9 in a dosage of 2 × 15 mg/kg/day. The combination of this treatment with fasting of the pregnant mice before and after the RA administration to increase the homogeneity of the response [23] resulted in systematic production of up to 13.5% of viable fetuses with TGA (Fig. 5). In subsequent studies with this specific treatment scheme the percentage rose to 64.3% (Fig. 6). This allowed us to proceed to the next phase of our studies, the stepwise analysis of the pathogenesis of TGA [42].

Table 4. Retinoic acid induced cardiac and extracardiac anomalies in fetal rats (Day 15 of gestation) 24 litters, 247 fetuses

	Day of administration							
Anomaly:	9.5	10	10.5	11	11.5	12	12.5	13
Cardiovascular								
TGA						1.2%		
PGA			21.0%	2.1%				
AoAA				4.2%	13.4%	32.0%		22.0%
DORV		18.2%	10.5%	43.8%	4.3%	43.9%		24.4%
VSD large			26.3%	12.5%				
VSD medium			5.2%	4.2%	43.8%	8.5%		6.7%
Extracardiac								
Exencephaly	50.0%	24.2%						
Spina bifida			27.3%	44.4%	12.5%			
Tail			10.5%	5.3%	60.4%	17.4%	23.8%	
Limbs		12.1%		10.4%		4.9%		80.0%
Face		31.5%		8.3%		1.2%		31.1%

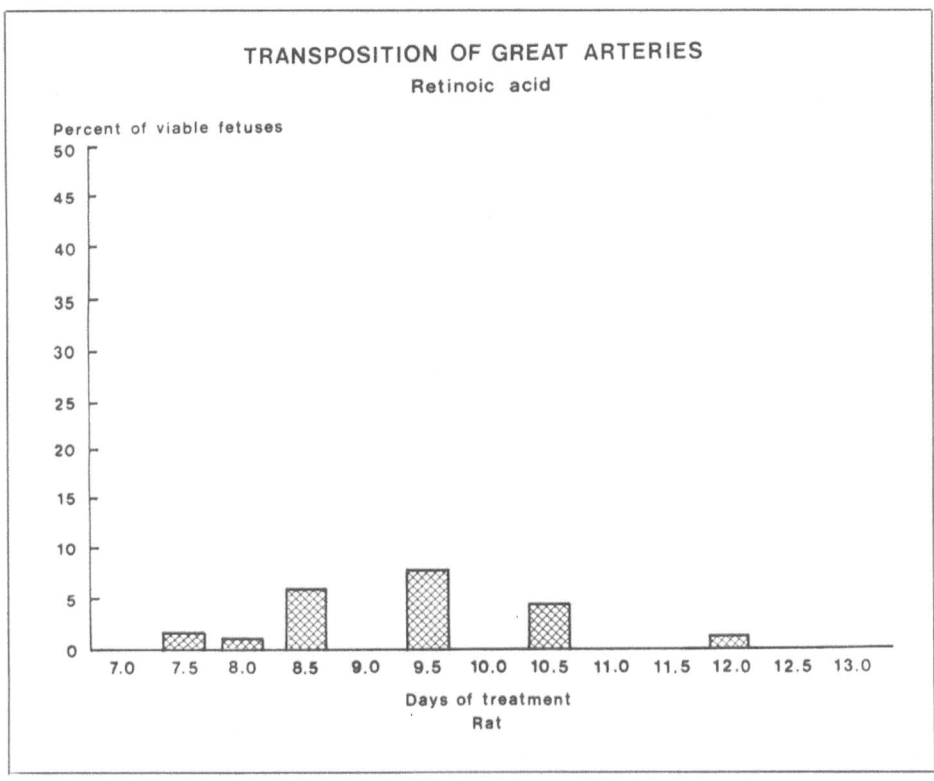

Fig. 4. Variation of incidence of TGA in Wistar rat embryos on gestation day 15 as a function of the day of retinoic acid administration

Stepwise analysis of TGA pathogenesis in RA exposed ICR mice

Between gestation days 11 (day of vaginal plug = day 1) and 15, the pregnant and treated ICR mice were sacrificed by cervical dislocation at 8 hours intervals. After removal of uterine horns, the embryos or fetuses were dissected free, perfusion fixed [31, 38], microdissected, and prepared for scanning electron microscopy, using a standardized procedure described previously [39]. Various steps of the microdissection were documented by photomacroscopy and scanning electron micrographs. Altogether, 304 embryos/fetuses were examined, using the above-mentioned procedures.

On day 11 of gestation, 48 h after the last RA administration, the very first change observed was abnormal looping of the heart (Fig. 7). From 19.1% of A- and L-loops discovered on that day their incidence rose to 72.5% on gestation day 14, with a shift from predominance of A-loops to L-loops. Twenty-four hours later, on day 12 of gestation, the conotruncus ridges were either not yet formed (25%) or were hypoplastic (75%), namely in their proximal portion (Fig. 8). Whereas in the normal embryos the aortico-pulmonary septum is present as early as gestation day

17

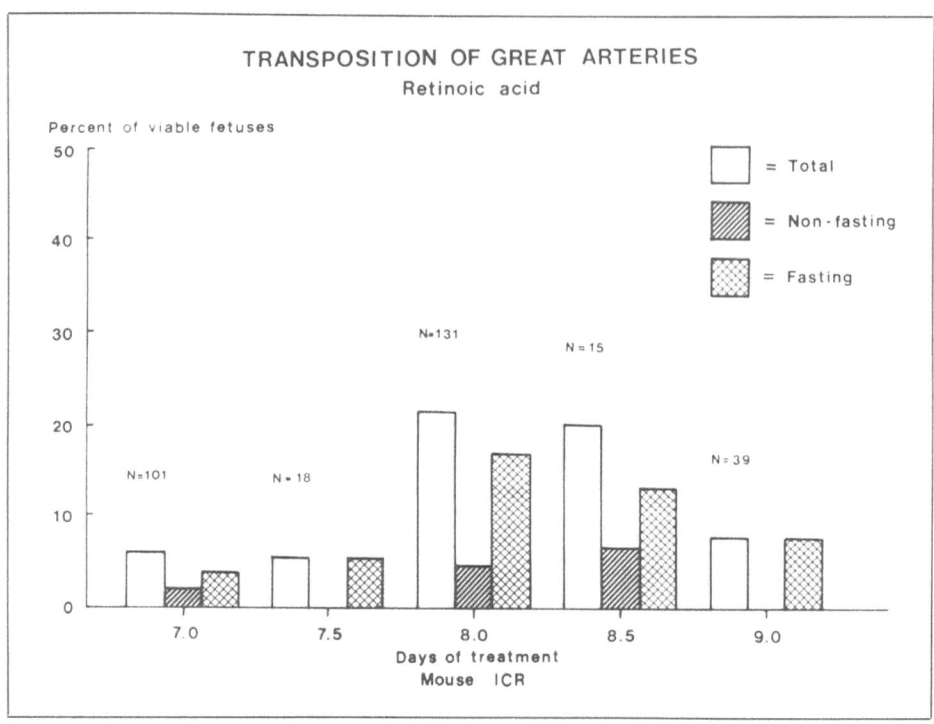

Fig. 5. Variation of incidence of TGA in ICR mouse embryos on gestation day 15, as a function of the day of retinoic acid administration and fasting

12, the treated embryos displayed a 40 h delay in formation of this structure. Despite this delay, its orientation was normal.

From the very beginning, the conotruncus ridges had an abnormal orientation, running parallel to each other on the ventral and dorsal faces of the conotruncus. Accessory ridges in the proximal portion of the conotruncus could be observed in up to 70% of abnormal embryos. Whereas the fusion of septal and parietal ridges normally starts after gestation day 12 plus 16 h, in treated embryos the first signs of a partial fusion were seen only from gestation day 13 plus 16 h onwards (Fig. 9). Complete fusion of these ridge was seen only on gestation day 16, with a delay of 40 h. Due to the hypoplasy of the proximal portion of the ridges, this fusion produced a short incomplete conotruncus septum. Interestingly, the formation of anlagen of semilunar valve cusps was not disturbed by the experimental intervention. On gestation day 13 plus 16 h the superior and inferior atrio ventricular (AV) cushions usually start their antero-posterior fusion. This fusion is delayed by 32 h (Fig. 9) in embryos exposed to RA, thus contributing to the persistence of the foramen interventriculare tertium which will persist as a ventricular septal defect (VSD) until delivery in at least half of the newborns (Fig. 10).

Table 5 summarizes the pathogenesis of TGA in this particular animal model: abnormal looping of the heart is followed by abnormal development of conotruncal

18

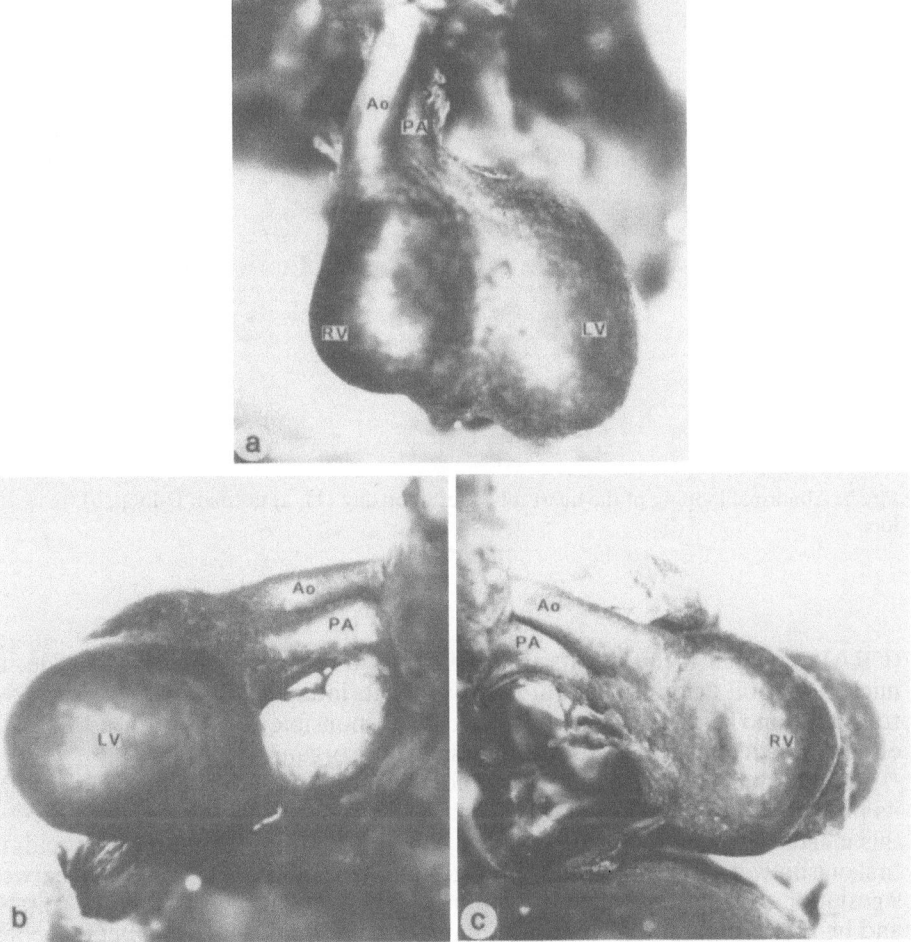

Fig. 6. TGA in ICR mouse embryo (gestation day 15), a) frontal, b) right profile, c) left profile views

ridges which will be hypoplastic and abnormally positioned. The aortico-pulmonary septum will have normal orientation, but its ingrowth and junction with the abnormal conotruncus ridges will be delayed. Delayed fusion of the AV-cushions will contribute to the final picture of TGA with (22.1%) or without (77.9%) VSD.

Interpretation, extrapolations, and conclusions

Let us first consider the mechanisms by which retinoic acid can interfere with cardiac development. All-trans retinoic acid or tretinoine, like other retinoids, pass across the cell membrane to be bound by cellular retinoic acid-binding protein

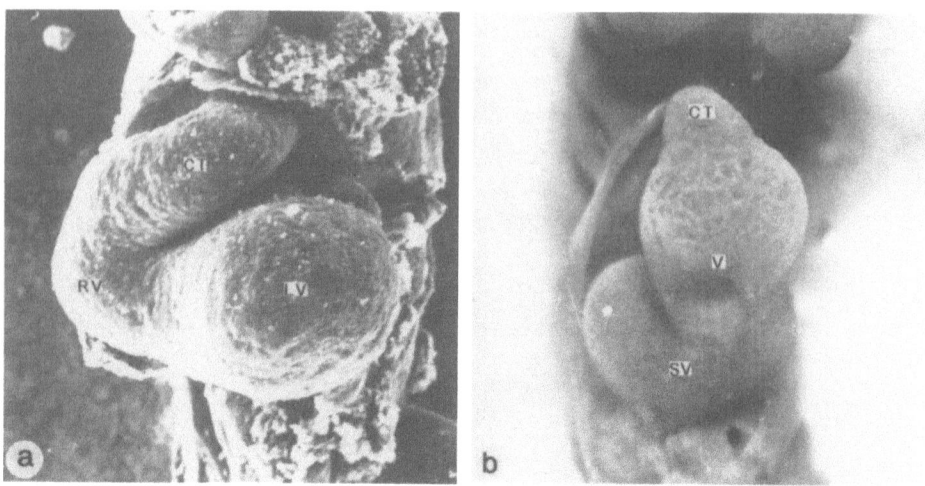

Fig. 7. Abnormal looping of the heart tube (gestation day 11), a) normal: D-loop, b) treated: A-loop

(CRABP) which facilitates its transfer across the nuclear envelope. Inside, the nuclear retinoic acid receptors are involved in its interactions with DNA and DNA transcription. It is this interaction which is responsible for the various biological effects known to affect almost every tissue in the organism.

The pharmacokinetic studies on retinoic acid in the pregnant mouse indicate that its plasmatic half-life is 6–10 h. Given the above mentioned treatment schedule, this means that the mouse embryos are exposed to two peaks of retinoic acid: the first one between 8 gestation days and 8 gestation days plus 12 h, the second between 9 gestation days and 9 gestation days plus 12 h. Investigations by Ruberte et al. [47] and by Dolle et al. [13] have shown that CRABP and retinoic acid beta receptors have a specific pattern of localization in embryonic tissues, a pattern which changes as the development progresses. These specific binding and receptor sites orient us about the parts of the embryonic body where the retinoic acid will exert its biological action. At the time of the first peak, CRABP was found in the cardiogenic plate and retinoic acid beta receptors in the adjacent mesenchyme. We speculate that it is during this very early period and at the binding sites mentioned that retinoic acid influences the heart tube formation, thus conditioning the subsequent abnormal looping of the heart. At the time of the second peak, retinoic acid gamma receptors were described in neural crest cells. From the work of Kirby's team [22], we know that cells derived from neural crest cells are involved in the development of the walls of the aortic arches and contribute to the aorticopulmonary septation. Without neglecting the potential role of modified hemodynamic of abnormally looped hearts, this effect on neural crest and their derivative might explain the delay in the ingrowth of the aortico-pulmonary septum, as well as the associated anomalies of aortic arches (19.4% of surviving embryos on gestation day 15).

How to explain the abnormal position and hypoplasy of the conotruncal ridges? Based on the extensive studies by Markwald and his team [27], we speculate that

20

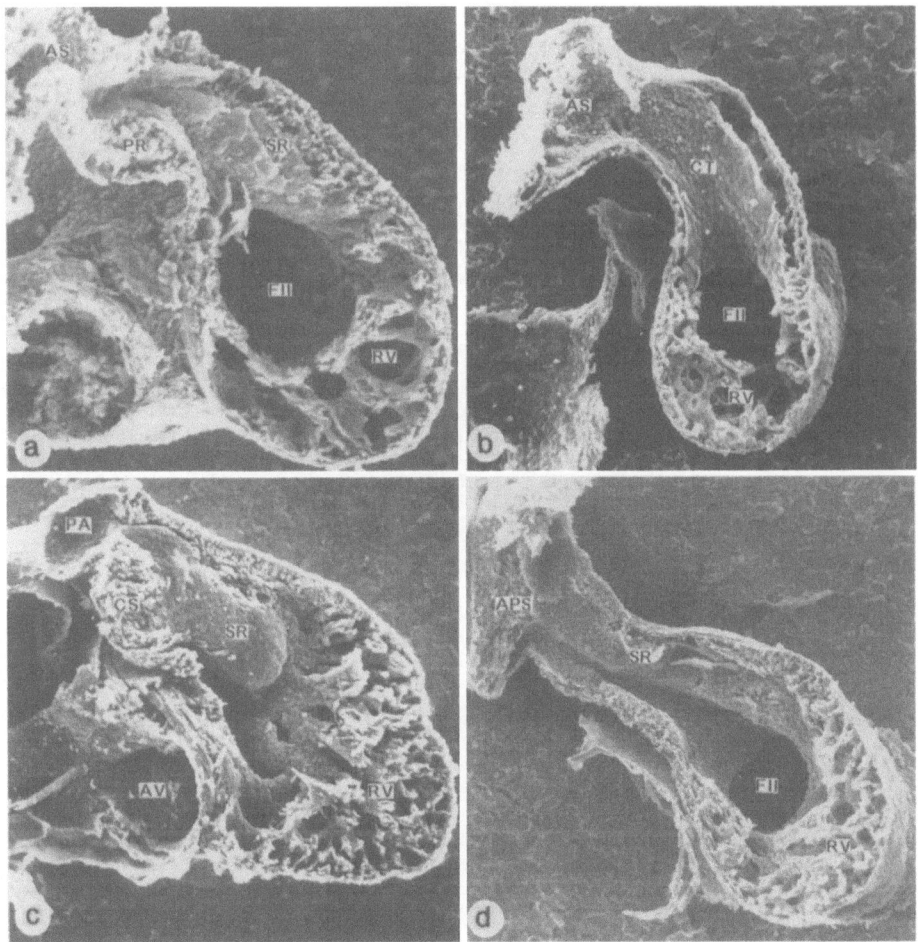

Fig. 8. Abnormal aortico-pulmonary and conotruncal septation: a) normal (gestation day (gd) 12), b) treated (12 gd). Note the complete absence of conotruncal ridges. c) normal (13 gd), spiralling septal ridge formed; d) treated (13 gd), deficient aortico-pulmonary septum, nonfused parallelly oriented conotruncal ridges

information about the formation of these ridges is encoded within the myocardium of the heart tube and is transmitted via the extracellular matrix of the cardiac jelly in the form of adherons towards the endocardium, in order to initiate seeding of the cardiac jelly ending with the formation of conotruncal ridges. Abnormal looping of the heart tube will displace the sites where these messengers initiate. A direct alteration of the messengers cannot yet be excluded. Other potential direct effects of retinoic acid on the extracellular matrix [35] or endothelial cells [7] have also to be considered.

Certain general rules operating during the pathogenesis of congenital heart disease were confirmed by these experiments: the relative independence of aortico-

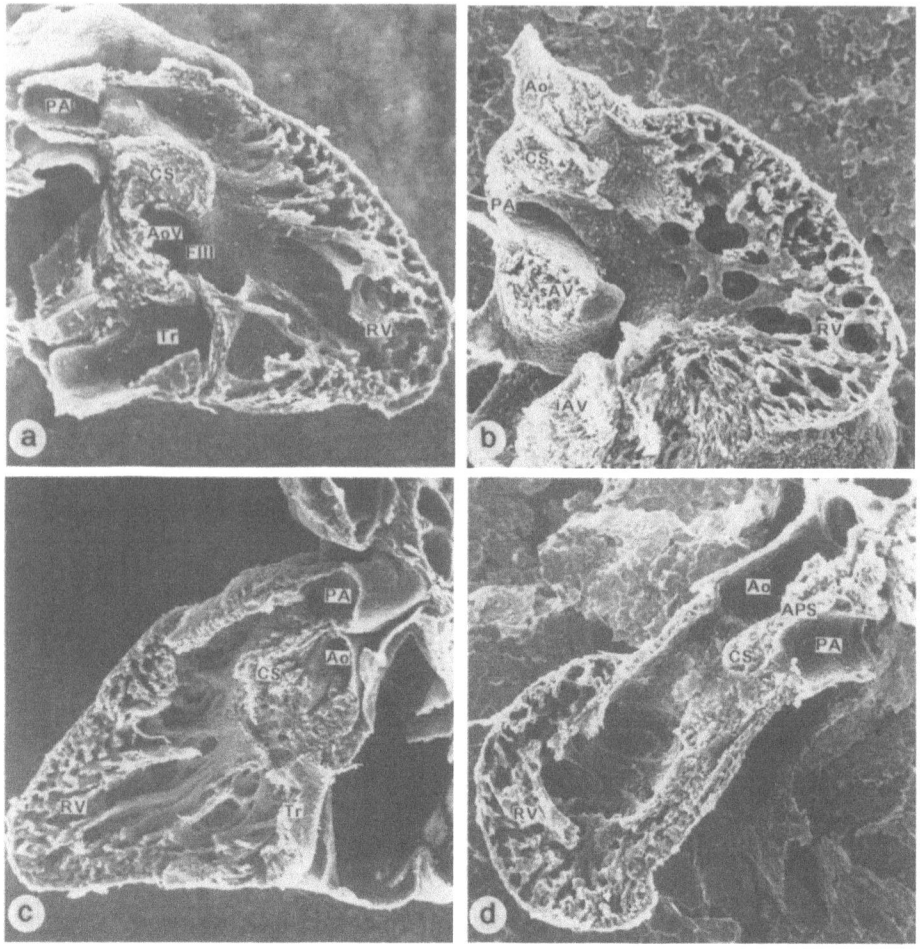

Fig. 9. Abnormal conotruncal septation: a) normal (14 gd) distal portion of the conotruncus septum formed, fused AV cushions; b) treated (14 gd) deficient distal portion of the conotruncus septum, nonfused AV cushions; c) normal (14 gd + 16 h) aortico-pulmonary and conotruncus septation completed; d) treated (14 gd + 16 h) absent conotruncus septum, completed aortico-pulmonary septation; abnormal position of the great arteries

pulmonary and conotruncal septation, the development of the semilunar valves from the distal portion of the conotruncal ridges, as well as the fact that some initial lesions (delayed fusion of the AV cushions) may no longer be visible in the malformed heart at delivery [40].

For a long time, TGA was considered by many authors as a conotruncal anomaly (Table 6). Our investigations indicate that, from the point of view of the site of primary impact and the initial phases of its pathogenesis, TGA is a looping and not a conotruncal anomaly. This is coherent with the epidemiological investigations [14], as well as with other experimental studies [15, 30, 43] indicating that TGA

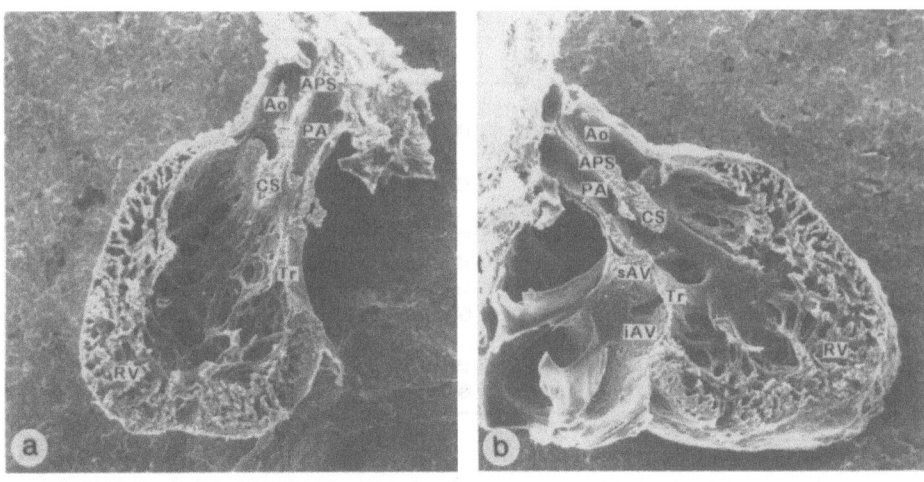

Fig. 10. D-TGA with AVSD (17 gd): a) normal aortico-pulmonary septum, rudimentary cono-truncus septum; b) atrioventricular septal defect (incompletely fused AV cushions) in subpulmonary location

Table 5. Pathogenesis of retinoic acid induced transposition of great arteries

Day of gestation	Normal	TGA
11	D-loop	A-loop
12	Spiralling conotruncus ridges	Parallel conotruncus ridges
13	Normal aortico-pulmonary septum	Hypoplastic aortico-pulmonary septum
	Conotruncus septum	Hypoplastic conotruncus ridges
14	Fusion of A-V cushions	Delayed fusion of AV-cushions
15	Normal heart	TGA + A-VSD

behaves differently from conotruncal anomalies, such as truncus arteriorus, pulmonary artery stenosis or atresia, double outlet right ventricle, and ventricular septal defects.

Further studies will be necessary to examine whether hitting the cardiogenic plate alone, without any interference with neural crest development, might also

23

Table 6. Conotruncal anomalies

Source	AoInt	TAC	TGA	TOF	PASt	PAAt	DORV	DOLV	VSD
Ivemark, 1955		●	●		●	●			
Van Praagh, 1973	●	●	●	●			●	●	
Angelini et al., 1974	●	●							
Fraser, Hunter, 1975			●	●	●				●
Patterson		●		●	●				●
Attie et al., 1979			●						
Miller, Smith, 1979			●	●	●	●			
Takao et al., 1980		●	●	●	●	●	●	●	
Hagler et al., 1980		●	●	●		●	●		●
Sanders et al., 1980		●	●	●		●			
Kouseff, 1984		●	●						
Shimizu et al., 1984	●	●	●	●		●			

produce this malformation. Experiments will be needed to verify the postulated mechanisms of interaction between retinoic acid and the developing heart.

Finally, we remind that our experimental studies may represent only one of many pathways which, in humans, results in the multitude of clinical forms of transposition of great arteries.

References

1. Anderson RH, Wilkinson J, Arnold R, Lubkiewitz K (1974) Morphogenesis of bulboventricular malformations. Br Heart J 36:242−256
2. Angelini P, Leachman RD (1974) Trunco-conal septal defects. An anatomic and embryologic discussion of common truncus and related malformations. Eur J Cardiol 2:11−22
3. Attie F, Kuri Alfaro J, Munoz Castellanos L, Arteaga M, Castro Bermudez A, Fernandez de la Vega P (1979) A study of the embryology of trunco-conal malformations. Arch Mal Coeur Vaiss 72:998−1005
4. Bankl H (1971) Mißbildungen des arteriellen Herzendes. Morphologie und Morphogenesis. Urban & Schwarzenberg, Wien
5. Bankl H (1972) Die Transposition der Herzostien. Ein Versuch ihrer Erklärung. Wien Klin Wochenschr 84:324−330
6. Barrow MV, Taylor WJ (1971) The production of congenital heart defects with the use of antisera to rat kidney, placenta and lung homogenates. Am Heart J 82:199−206
7. Braunhut SJ, Palomares M (1991) Modulation of endothelial cell shape and growth by retinoids. Microvasc Res 41:47−62
8. Chuaqui B (1979) Doerr's theory of morphogenesis of arterial transposition in light of recent research. Br Heart J 41:481−485
9. Chuaqui B, Bersch W (1973) The formal genesis of the transposition of great arteries. Virch Arch [A] 358:11−34
10. Conte G (1976) Ulteriore Contributo alla Conoscenza dell'ontogenesi della "Transposizione completa delle grosse arterie del cuore" (A further contribution to the ontogenesis of "Complete Transposition" of the great arteries) Atti della Societa Italiana di Anatomia: XXXIII Convegno Nazionale in Catania, 22−25 settembre
11. Conte G, Arrigioni P (1966) Precisazioni Embriologiche su Due Alterazioni Congenite di Prima Formazione del Cuore: Aorta a Cavaliere e Transposizione Completa dei Grossi Vasi.

Estratto da: Atti del XXVII Cong. della Soc. Ital. di Cardiologia. Sirmione 2−5 Giugno. Vol II. Il Pensiere Scientifico, ed. Roma

12. Davis LA, Sadler TW (1980) Effects of vitamin A on development of endocardial cushions. Anat Rec 196:42A−43A
13. Dolle P, Ruberte E, Leroy P, Morriss-Kay G, Chambon LP (1990) Retinoic acid receptors and cellular retinoid binding proteins: 1. A systematic study of their differential pattern of transcription during mouse organogenesis. Development 110:1133−1151
14. Ferencz C, Rubin JD, McCarter RJ, Boughman JA, Wilson PD, Brenner JI, Neill CA, Perry LW, Hepner SI, Downing JW (1987) Cardiac and noncardiac malformations: observations in a population-based study. Teratology 35:367−378
15. Fox MH, Goss CM (1956) Experimental production of a syndrome of congenital cardiovascular defects in rats. Anat Rec 124:189−207
16. Fraser FC, Hunter ADW (1975) Etiologic relations among categories of congenital heart malformations. Am J Cardiol 36:793−796
17. Hagler DJ, Tajik AI, Seward JB, Mair DD, Ritter DG (1980) Wide-angle two-dimensional echocardiographic profiles of conotruncal abnormalities. Mayo Clin Proc 55:73−82
18. Haring OM (1966) Cardiac malformations in the rat induced by maternal hypercapnia with hypoxia. Circ Res 19:544−551
19. Irie K, Ando M, Takao A (1990) All-Trans retinoic acid induced cardio-vascular malformations. In: Bockman DE, Kirby ML (eds) Embryonic Origins of Defective Heart Development. N Y Acad Sci, New York, pp 387−388
20. Ivemark BI (1955) Implications of agenesis of the spleen on the pathogenesis of cono-truncal anomalies in childhood: Analysis of heart malformations in splenic agenesis syndrome, with 14 new cases. Acta paediat (Uppsala) Suppl. 104, 44:1−110
21. Khera KS, Heggtveit MA (1974) Fetal cardiovascular defects induced by thalidomide in the cat. Teratology 9:A-24
22. Kirby ML, Waldo KL (1990) Role of neural crest in congenital heart disease. Circulation 82:332−340
23. Koshar D (1989) personal communication
24. Kousseff BG (1984) Sacral meningocele with conotruncal heart defects − A possible autosomal recessive trait. Pediatrics 74:385−398
25. Lev M, Saphir O (1945) A theory of transposition of the arterial trunks based on the phylogenetic and ontogenetic development of the heart. Arch Pathol 39:172−183
26. Losekoot TG, Anderson RH, Becker AE, Danielson GK, Soto B (1983) Congenitally corrected transposition. Churchill Livingstone, Edinburgh
27. Markwald RR, Mjaatvedt CH, Krug EL, Sinning AR (1990) Inductive interactions in heart development: Role of cardiac adherons in cushion tissue formation. In: Bockman DE, Kirby ML (eds) Embryonic Origins of Defective Heart Development. N Y Acad Sci, New York, pp 13−25
28. Miller PD, Telford IR, Haas GR (1971) Effect of hyperbaric oxygen on cardiogenesis in the rat. Biol Neonate 17:44−52
29. Miller ME, Smith DW (1979) Conotruncal malformation complex − Examples of possible monogenic inheritance. Pediatrics 63:890−893
30. Monie IW, Takacs E, Warkany J (1966) Transposition of the great vessels and other cardiovascular abnormalities in rat fetuses induced by trypan blue. Anat Rec 156:175−190
31. Moscoso G, Pexieder T (1990) Variations in microscopic anatomy and ultrastructure of human embryonic hearts subjected to three different modes of fixation. Path Res Pract 186:768−774
32. Okamoto N (1976) Morphogenesis of the transposition of the great vessels. Cong Anom 16:129−145
33. Okamoto N, Satow Y, Hidaka N, Akimoto N, Miyabara S (1978) Morphogenesis of congenital heart anomaly − bulboventricular malformations. Jap Circ J 42:1105−1120
34. Orts-Llorca F, Domenech Mateu JM, Puerta-Fonolla J (1983) Transposicion tipica completa de los grandes arterias (TGA) en un embrion humano de 19 mm. Uno nueva teoria sobre su embriogenesis. Rev Espan Cardiol 36:81−88
35. Paige K, Palomares M, D'Amore PA, Braunhut SJ (1991) Retinol-induced modification of the extracellular matrix of endothelial cells: its role in growth control. In Vitro Cell Dev Biol 27A:151−157

36. Patterson DF (1978) Lesion-specific genetic factors in canine congenital heart disease: patent ductus arteriosus in poodles, defects of the conotruncal septum in the Keeshond. In: Rosenquist GC, Bergsma D (eds) Morphogenesis and Malformation of the Cardiovascular System. Birth Defects: Orig. Art. Ser., Vol XIV N° 7. Alan R. Liss Inc (New York), pp 345–347

37. Pernkopf E, Wirtinger W (1935) Das Wesen der Transposition im Gebiete des Herzens, ein Versuch der Erklärung auf entwicklungsgeschichtlicher Grundlage. Virchows Arch 295:143–175

38. Pexieder T (1981) Prenatal development of the endocardium: a review. Scanning Electron Microscopy II:223–253

39. Pexieder T (1986) Standardized method for study of normal and abnormal cardiac development in chick, rat, mouse, dog and human embryos. Teratology 33:91C

40. Pexieder T (1981) Cellular abnormalities leading to congenital heart disease. In: Goodman M (ed) Paediatric Cardiology, vol. 4. Churchill Livingstone, Edinburgh, pp 24–32

41. Pexieder T, Bloch D, Beuret A (1989) Eurocat collaborative study on congenital heart disease. Eur J Epidemiol 5:254

42. Pexieder T, Pfizenmaier Rousseil M (1991) Pathogenesis of retinoic acid induced transposition of great arteries. Circulation 84:II–385

43. Pexieder T, Pfizenmaier Rousseil M, Prados Frutos JC (1990) Spectrum of cardiac and extracardiac anomalies induced by retinoic acid in rats. Teratology 41:584

44. Pexieder T, Vuillemin M, Alaili R, Veuthy S, Patterson DF, Scott WJ Jr. (1989) Experimental studies in the pathogenesis of conotruncal defects. In: Aranega A, Pexieder T (eds) Correlation between Experimental Cardiac Embryology and Teratology and Congenital Cardiac Defects. University of Granada, Granada, pp 37–92

45. Pohanka I, Vítek B (1972) Survey of embryology of the heart and the most important pathogenetic theories of great vessel transposition. Cesk Patol 17:8–16

46. Robertson J (1913) The comparative anatomy of the bulbus cordis with special reference to abnormal positions of the great vessel in the human heart. J Pathol Bact 18:191–210

47. Ruberte E, Dolle P, Krust A, Zelent A, Morriss-Kay G, Chambon P (1990) Specific spatial and temporal distribution of retinoic acid receptor gamma transcripts during mouse embryogenesis. Development 108:213–222

48. Sanders SP, Bierman FZ, Williams RG (1982) Conotruncal malformations – diagnosis in infancy using subxiphoid 2-dimensional echocardiography. Am J Cardiol 50:1361–1367

49. Shaner RF (1962) Comparative development of the bulbus and ventricles of the vertebrate heart with special reference to Spitzer's theory of heart malformations. Anat Rec 142:519–529

50. Shimizu T, Takao A, Ando M, Hirayama A (1984) Conotruncal anomaly face syndrome: its heterogeneity and association with thymus involution. In: Nora JJ, Takao A (eds) Congenital Heart Disease. Causes and Processes. Futura Publ. Co, Mount Kisco, N.Y., pp 29–42

51. Sonoda T, Ohdo S, Ohba KI, Okishima T, Hayakawa K (1991) Sodium valproate-induced cardiovascular abnormalities in the Jcl:ICR mouse fetus. Cong Anom 31:89–94

52. Steding G, Seidl W (1984) Zur Entwicklung der Transpositionen der großen Gefäße. Verh Anat Ges 78:263–264

53. Sukumar IP (1976) A new look at transposition of great arteries. J Ass Phys India 24:531–533

54. Takao A, Ando M, Cho K, Kinouchi A, Murakami Y (1980) Etiologic categorization of common congenital disease. In: Van Praagh R, Takao A (eds) Etiology and Morphogenesis of Congenital Heart Disease. Futura Publ Co, Mount Kisco, N.Y., pp 253–269

55. Taylor IM, Agur A, Wiley MJ (1978) Retinoic acid-induced malformation of the heart. J Anat 127:646

56. Ueno T (1973) The association of sulpho-mucopolysaccharides with histogenesis of endocardial swellings (cushion tissues) in normal and abnormal developing rat heart. Med J Hiroshima Univ 21:619–644

57. Van Mierop LHS, Wiglesworth FW (1963) Pathogenesis of transposition complexes. III True transposition of the great vessels. Am J Cardiol 12:233–239

58. Van Praagh R (1973) Transposition des gros vaisseaux: définition, historique et corrélation anatomo-radiologiques. Coeur 4:207–228

59. Vickers TH (1968) The cardiovascular malformations in the rabbit thalidomide embryopathy. Br Exp Pathol 49:149–196

60. Von Rokitansky C (1875) Die Defekte der Scheidewände des Herzens. Wilhelm Braumüller, Wien
61. Vuillemin M, Pexieder T (1989) Normal stages of cardiac organogenesis in the mouse. II. Development of the internal relief of the heart. Am J Anat 184:114−128

Author's address:
T. Pexieder, M.D.
Institut d'Histologie et d'Embryologie
Université de Lausanne
Rue du Bugnon 9
1005 Lausanne
Suisse

Development of coronary arteries in transposition of the great arteries

A. C. Gittenberger-de Groot, R. E. Poelmann, R. Bökenkamp[1], A. J. J. C. Bogers[2]
[1]Department of Anatomy and Embryology, University of Leiden,
The Netherlands
[2]Department of Thoracic Surgery, Thoraxcenter, University of Rotterdam,
The Netherlands

Introduction

The study of the origin and branching pattern of the coronary arteries in transposition of the great arteries (TGA) needs updating. A thorough investigation of all variations has been documented [12], but it lacks the special emphasis that would make it relevant for present clinical use. This latter subject refers to the arterial-switch operation in which the main procedure for surgical correction of TGA is performed at the level of the great arteries [7]. An essential part is the feasibility of surgical relocation of the coronary arteries to the newly formed aortic orifice, being originally the pulmonary orifice. The former classification of the coronary arterial origin was far too complicated to be able to sort out which type of coronary arterial pattern could be switched and in which cases it would be wiser to develop an alternative technique or to stay with the already well-known Mustard or Senning procedures.

An important hinderance to the study proved to be the classical nomenclature for the semilunar valves of both the aorta and pulmonary orifice. This terminology is positional in nature, referring to right, left, and posterior sinuses. With the variable relationship of the aortic and pulmonary orifice in TGA this led to a misleading high number of variations in origin and branching pattern. The simplification of this system will be described in the next section.

For our study, 103 cases of TGA from the Leiden collection of post-mortem specimens with congenital heart disease were available. These were classified and restudied with the help of the pediatric cardiologist Ursula Sauer and the thoracic surgeon Jan Quaegebeur (see chapters by them in this volume). The results of this anatomical study will be discussed in the present chapter.

The last part of this chapter will deal in more detail with our current research of the normal and abnormal development of the coronary arteries in general.

Terminology

In classical terminology of the heart the semilunar sinuses of the arterial orifices are named after their position in the body. For the present study the nomenclature for the aortic orifice is the most important. The right semilunar sinus bears the origin of

Supported by grants from the Deutsche Forschungsgemeinschaft and the Netherlands Organization for Scientific Research (NWO)

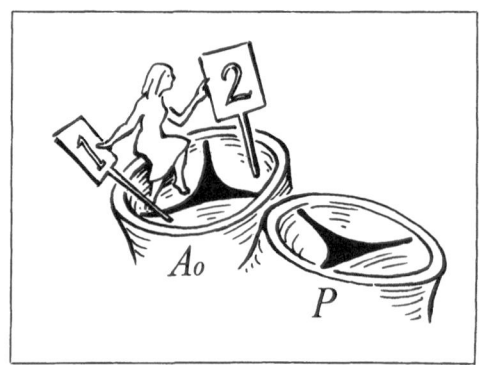

Fig. 1. Schematic representation of the aortic (Ao) and pulmonary (P) orifice. If one takes the position in the non-facing (non-coronary) cusp of the aortic valve, the righthand sinus is referred to as sinus 1 and the lefthand sinus as sinus 2

the right coronary artery, whereas the left gives rise to the left coronary artery. The non-coronary cusp is referred to as such, or is called the posterior sinus. In adult cardiology and in congenital malformation in which the relative postion of the pulmonary and aortic orifice is not critical this terminology is simple. However, if the aorta, as is typical for transposition, comes into a side-to-side, right anterior, frontal or left anterior position relative to the pulmonary orifice, complications arise. The semilunar sinuses change their positional name. This aspect has been described earlier [4]. The solution turned out to be a nomenclature that was based on a stable relationship of the aortic and pulmonary orifice, independent of their position in the body. In normal development two facing sinuses in each orifice are present that actually face the other orifice. If the pulmonary orifice is considered as a fixed point, the aortic orifice can circle around. The two facing sinuses, however, will always be directed towards the pulmonary orifice. It was then decided that, viewed from the non-facing (non-coronary) sinus, the aortic sinus on the righthand side would be called sinus 1 and the facing sinus on the lefthand side sinus 2 (Fig. 1). For "everyday" use the term righthand sinus and lefthand sinus are practical. If data on coronary arterial origin are stored in automatic database systems the description of the various types is more efficient when 1 and 2 are used for naming of the sinuses.

Simplifying the system further, it was recognized that the right and left coronary arteries and their variations were considered to be built-up of three major branches. These are the right coronary artery (RCA, or R), the left anterior descending artery (LAD, or L) and the left circumflex artery (LCx, or Cx). The various arteries can either originate separately or in any combination from sinus 1 and/or 2, with only one common orifice or from separate orifices. The non-facing sinus is essentially non-coronary in nature. Sometimes an accessory branch can arise separately and additional to one of the three main branches; it is usually small and does not follow an extensive course.

A rule that relates to the course of the coronary arteries is that they never cross each other.

Combination of a new nomenclature for the semilunar sinuses and the recognition of three main arterial branches has led to a major simplification of the coronary

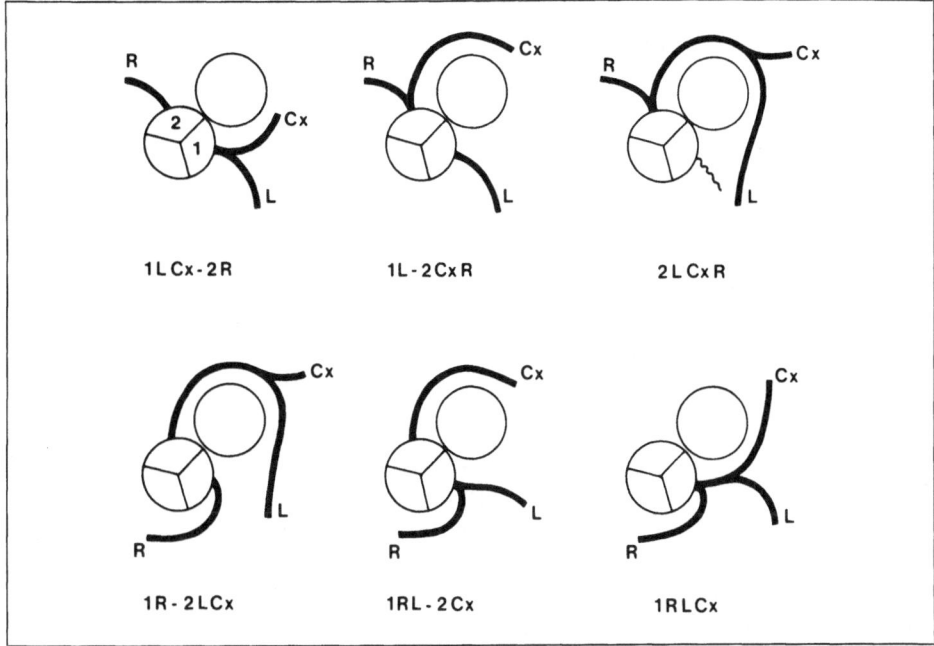

Fig. 2. The six main types of coronary arterial origin and branching pattern in TGA. R: right coronary artery; L: left anterior descending artery; Cx: left circumflex artery. Four variations show a dual origin of the coronary arteries, which thus arise from sinuses 1 and 2. In the last cases of the top and bottom row there is a single sinus origin. If more than one main branch originates from a sinus there can be one or two orifices. (Figure taken from [10])

arterial pattern, based essentially on six main types. This has been advocated by Anderson [1] as the Leiden convention.

Variation in origin and branching pattern in TGA

For TGA the results of the simplification of the classification will be described first at the level of variation in origin (Fig. 2). It shows the basic principle of the six main types, four of which have a dual origin of the coronary arteries using both the right-hand (1) and the lefthand sinus (2), and two types in which all arterial supply is derived from one sinus. It is important to note that not all variations are equally common. Figure 3 shows the predominance of 1:L,Cx-2:R, followed by 1:L-2:CxR. It is also obvious that the relative positions of the aortic and pulmonary orifices influences the pattern that is found. The most common pattern is clearly related to a right anterior position of the aorta. Far more variability is seen if the aortic and pulmonary orifices are in a side-to-side relationship. A phenomenon that is not shown in detail in this chapter is the variation in the proximal course. The most variable cases are found in a side-to-side relationship. The variations have been extensively described [4, 10]. A common rule that might facilitate the understanding of this finding is that, in general, the coronary arteries tend to take the shortest course

31

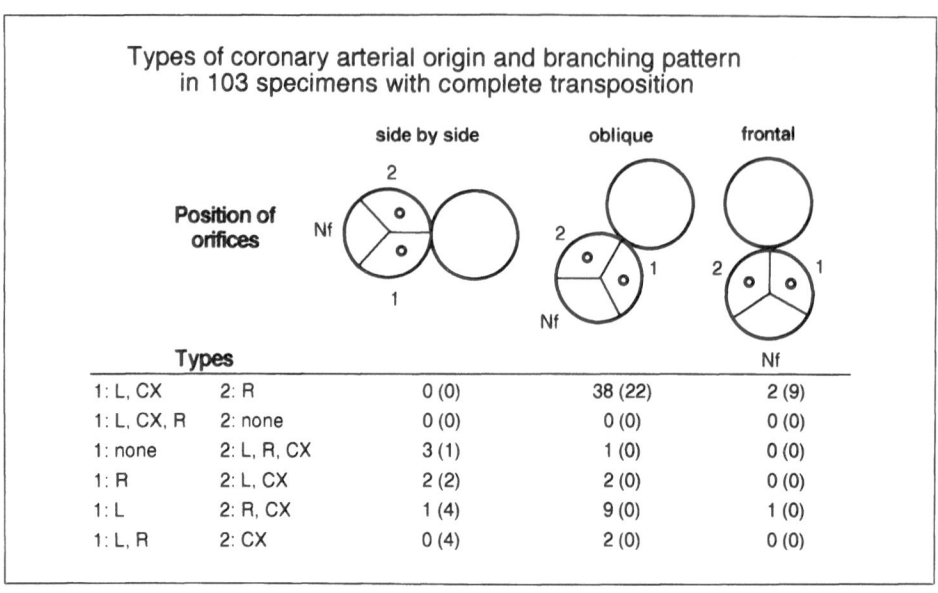

Fig. 3. Variations in origin and branching pattern in TGA correlated with the relative position of the aortic and pulmonary orifice. The cases in brackets indicate the cases of TGA with a ventricular septal defect

towards their interventricular or atrioventricular sulcus. The work of Quaegebeur [10] has shown a slight difference in results because of a small positional shift. Obviously, the opinion of a surgeon as to what is side-to-side, right anterior, and frontal is a bit different. The main message, however, is not altered.

Consequences for the choice of surgery

The above results were carefully evaluated by the thoracic surgeon Quaegebeur, as to their possible hazards during the performance of the arterial switch procedure. Morphology and statistical analysis showed that, essentially, only one variation in coronary arterial anatomy proved to be hazardous [5]. These are cases with a so-called aortic intramural coronary artery. The three cases that were originally found among the 103 cases tend to give a good indication of the frequency in which this anomaly occurs. Visual inspection of the outer aspect of the base of the heart is misleading. Figure 4 shows the most common form of origin of the left anterior descending and the circumflex artery from sinus 1. This artery can easily be translocated to its new site in the facing sinus of the pulmonary orifice. Figure 5 shows a case which, upon cursory inspection seems to have the right coronary artery and the left anterior descending artery arising from sinus 1, whereas the circumflex arises from sinus 2. In fact, all arteries arise from sinus 2. A similar case with a different branching pattern is presented schematically in Fig. 6. This shows the problem that the coronary artery shares the media of its wall with the aorta. In two of the three cases the orifice was very typically located just behind a commissure and it was slit-

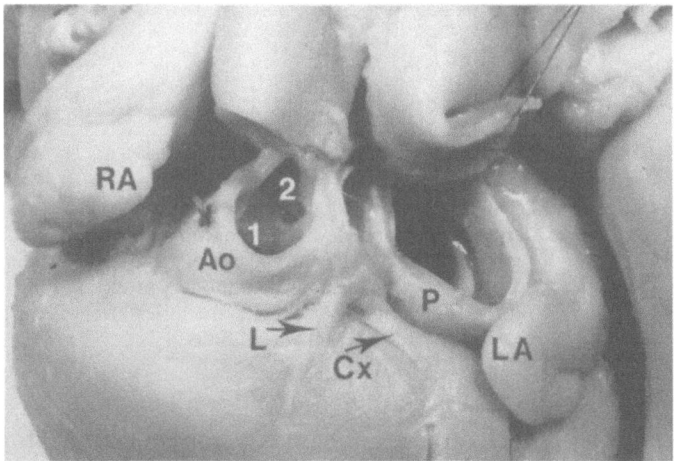

Fig. 4. Frontal view of a specimen with TGA. This case presents with the most common form of branching pattern. The left anterior descending (L) and the left circumflex (Cx) arise from sinus 1 of the aorta (Ao). Sinus is 2 seen as well. Pulmonary artery: P; right atrium: RA; left atrium: LA

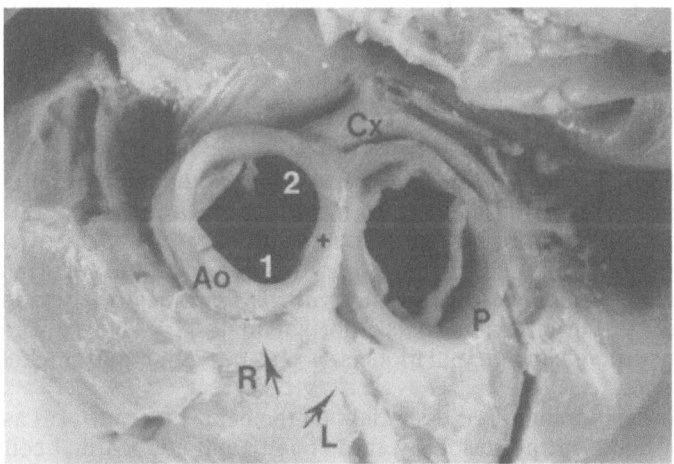

Fig. 5. Coronary arterial branching pattern in TGA in a case with an aortic intramural course of a coronary artery. The right coronary artery (R) and the left anterior descending (L) run partly in the aortic wall (+) and originate from sinus 2, like the circumflex artery (Cx) which takes a course posterior to the pulmonary orifice (P). (Figure taken from [5])

like in form. In these cases the coronary artery cannot be mobilized by the surgeon in the usual way. Alternative surgical approaches have been described [10].

This brings us to the last aspect of the clinical consequences that refers to the diagnostics available before surgery, and which might indicate beforehand what type of origin and branching pattern might be expected. At present, angiocardiography [11] is only of limited use, because an aortic intramural course cannot be detected with this method. Occasional accounts of successful detection by echocar-

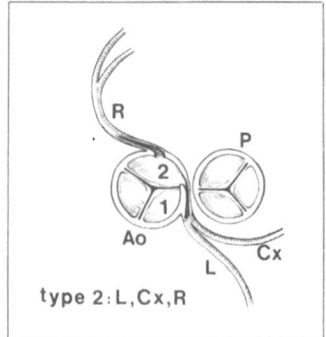

type 2: L,Cx,R

Fig. 6. Schematic view of a case with an aortic intramural coronary artery. The coronary artery shares the media of the aortic wall. Aorta: Ao; pulmonary artery: P; left anterior descending artery: L; circumflex artery Cx; right coronary artery: R; sinus 1: 1; sinus 2: 2

diography have been reported. Mostly, these are based on a specific search for a possible intramural course. An indication for this type of special diagnostic emphasis might be given to those cases with a side-to-side origin of the great arteries, as these tend to have the highest variation in origin and branching pattern.

At the least, the surgeon should always check the site of origin by viewing the orifices from above after dissecting the great arteries. The possibility of high take-off should be taken into account as a variation that is regularly seen. It was found in one of the three cases with aortic intramural course [4, 5].

Development aspects

The above-described stability of coronary arterial origin with regard to their relationship to the facing aortic semilunar sinuses, combined with a comparable stability of the arteries in their more peripheral course in the various sulci of the heart, as well as the instability of the proximal course in the area of the aortic and pulmonary orifice seems a challenge for the embryologist. Classical theories on development of coronary arterial orifices were not adequate [2]. Therefore, an appropriate study was started using animal models such as rat, quail, and chicken-quail chimeras.

In coronary vascular development it is essential that the heart tube starts off as a nude myocardial tube lined on the inside by cardiac jelly and endocardial cells. Only secondarily is this heart tube covered by an epicardial layer. This epicardium derives from an outgrowth of the epicardial organ, consisting of bleb-like protrusions (Fig. 7). This epicardial organ originates from the coelomic wall in the area of the septum transversum and liver in mammals and, as birds do not posses a transverse septum, from the liver region in birds (Fig. 7). The development of the epicardium has been described [6], but has not been related to the development of the coronary vascular system. Our most recent results show that the epicardial blebs spread over the surface of the heart starting from the inner curvature and, last of all, covering the lateral aspects of the ventricles. The first endothelial cells necessary for the development of the coronary vessels follow soon after. Initially they were thought to develop from the epicardium itself [13], but our chicken-quail chimera experiments have conclusively shown that there is an invasion of the sub-epicardial space by endothelial cells that arises from the liver region. Very essential

34

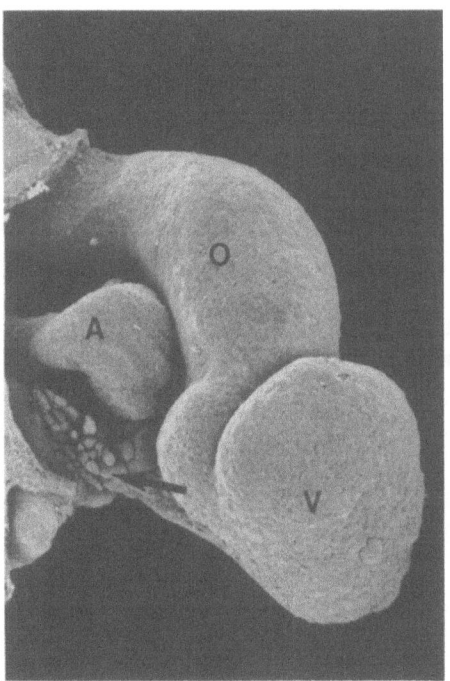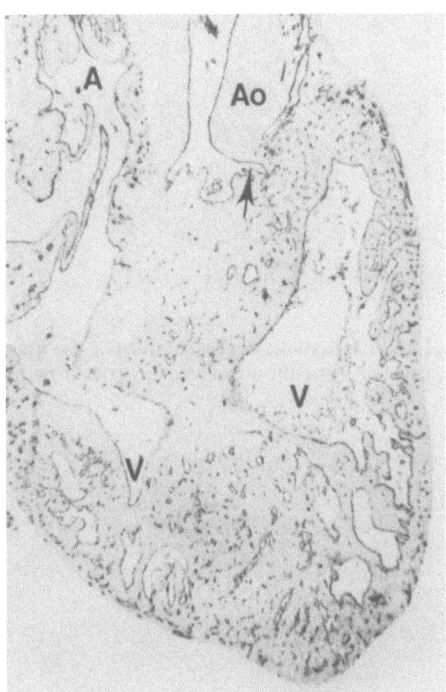

Fig. 7. Scanning electron micrograph of a quail heart of 5 days' development. The apex of the ventricle (V) has been somewhat tilted to expose the bleb-like protrusions of the epicardial organ (arrow). Outflow tract: O; atrium: A

Fig. 8. Section of a quail heart of 7 days' development. There is extensive staining of the endocardial lining of the ventricles (V) and atria (A). The elastic media of the aortic wall (Ao) is devoid of vessels except for one coronary artery (arrow). The subepicardial coronary arteries have invaded the myocardial wall. Staining with a specific antibody (MB1) against quail endothelial cells [18]

was the availability of a specific antibody against quail endothelial cells [8]. With this technique it is possible to stain every endothelial cell, but also every endocardial cell of the quail (Fig. 8).

The results can be summarized as follows. The endothelial cells spread initially as isolated cells over the surface of the heart, with a marked preference for the atrioventricular and interventricular regions. In the present work, we will emphasize the connection with the arterial orifice level. Figure 8 shows that the arterial wall of the great vessels is not yet vascularized, thus allowing for a detailed study of the development of the origin of the coronary arteries related to the semilunar sinuses. In work from our group by Bogers et al. [3], it has been shown that we are not dealing with an outgrowth of the coronary arteries from the aortic orifice, but with an ingrowth into the aortic wall (Fig. 9). This phenomenon has been unequivocally substantiated by chicken-quail chimera experiments (Fig. 10). In these experiments a small piece of quail liver is transplanted in the pericardial cavity of the chick [9]. It adheres to the myocardial wall. The endothelial cells of

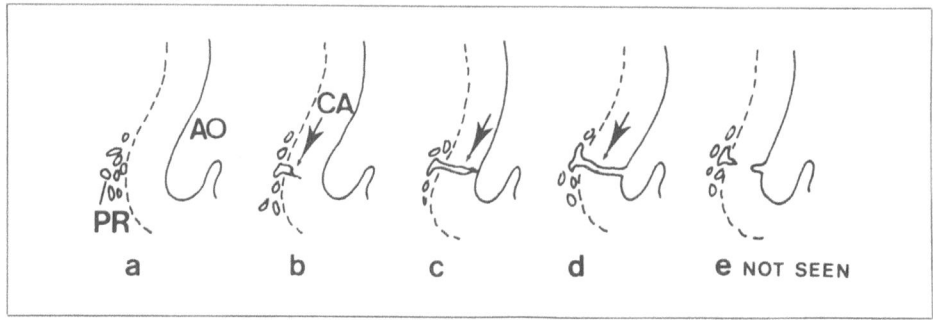

Fig. 9. Schematic representation of the ingrowth of a coronary artery (CA) from the peritruncal ring (PR) into the aorta (Ao). An outgrowth (panel e) has not been found. (Figure taken from [3])

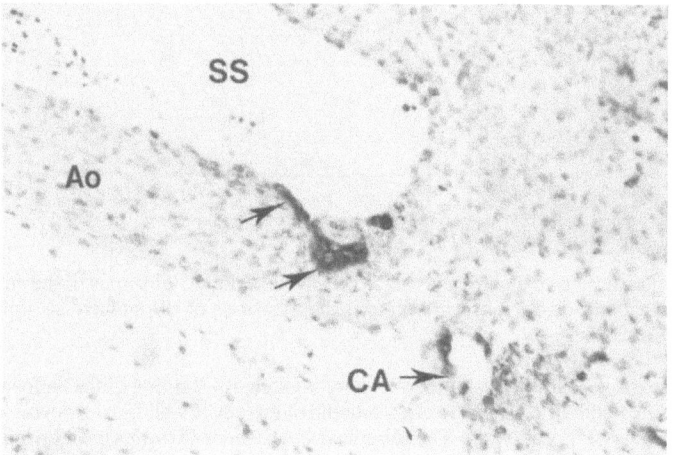

Fig. 10. Section through a facing semilunar sinus (SS) of the aortic orifice in a chicken-quail chimera. The dark staining (MB1) endothelial cells (arrows) of the quail are lining part of a coronary artery (CA) and have moved through the aortic wall (Ao) to the endothelial lining of the sinus, which is of chicken origin

the quail are recruited for the normal development of the coronary vessels of the chick. Additionally, the quail cells can be detected specifically by the antibody, showing that, indeed, the coronary arterial endothelial cells invade the aortic wall.

Our current research concentrates on the factors that are responsible for the specific ingrowth sites. It is still not clear what actually dictates the stable ingrowth pattern in the two facing semilunar sinuses of the aorta. The situation has become even more complicated as it has been shown that the aortic orifice has more sites of ingrowth of endothelial cells (i.e., also in the third non-facing sinus) while only two of these endothelial strands in the facing sinuses actually luminize.

The pulmonary orifice is devoid of ingrowth sites under normal circumstances. The interest now focuses on the origin and timing of the formation of the peritruncal ring of endothelial cells encircling the arterial orifice level. In the work of Bogers et al. this was shown schematically to be a saddle-shaped outer ring [3]. From this band of endothelial cells, one could easily deduct the possible variations in proximal course. The course of a coronary artery in-between the aortic and pulmonary orifice was, however, not accounted for. Three-dimensional reconstructions of this area have shown that the saddle-shaped ring, in fact, consists of two interconnected rings, which does allow an explanation for arteries that run in-between the aortic and pulmonary orifice. It also shows that the aortic orifice is encircled earlier as compared to the pulmonary orifice. Further research is still necessary to explain the mechanism of selective ingrowth into the facing aortic semilunar sinuses. Most probably, we have to solve at a more basic level the point of what actually defines an aorta and distinguishes it from the adjoining pulmonary artery. This question also bears relevance for our general understanding of development of TGA.

References

1. Anderson RH, Henry W, Becker AE (1991) Morphologic aspects of complete transposition. Cardiol Young 1:41–53
2. Bogers AJJC, Gittenberger-de Groot AC, Dubbeldam JA, Huysmans HA (1988) The inadequacy of existing theories on development of the proximal coronary arteries and their connections with the arterial trunks. Int J Cardiol 20:117–123
3. Bogers AJJC, Gittenberger-de Groot AC, Poelmann RE, Peault BM, Huysmans HA (1989) Development of the origin of the coronary arteries, a matter of ingrowth or outgrowth. Anat Embryol 180:437–441
4. Gittenberger-de Groot AC, Sauer U, Quaegebeur J (1983) Coronary arterial anatomy in transposition of the great arteries: A morphologic study. Pediatr Cardiol 4 (Suppl):I 15–24
5. Gittenberger-de Groot AC, Sauer U, Quaegebeur JM (1986) Aortic intramural coronary artery in three hearts with transposition of the great arteries. J Thorac Cardiovasc Surg 91:566–571
6. Ho E, Shimada Y (1978) Formation of the epicardium studied with the scanning electron microscope. Dev Biol 66:579–585
7. Kirklin JW (1991) The surgical repair for complete transposition. Cardiol Young 1:13–25
8. Peault BM (1987) MB1, a quail leukocyte/vascular endothelium antigen: characterization of the lymphocyte-surface form and identification of its secreted counterpart as alpha-2-macroglobulin. Cell Differ 23:165–174
9. Poelmann RE, Gittenberger-de Groot AC, Mentink MMT, De Ruiter MC, Groot E, Hoedemaeker R, Coltey M, Christ B (1990) Endothelial cell migration in the developing blood vessel system of chicken/quail chimaeras. Eur J Cell Biol 53 (Suppl 31):48–49
10. Quaegebeur JM (1986) The arterial switch operation. Rationale, results, perspectives. Thesis, Leiden. Uitg. Rozengaard-Deerlijk, Belgie
11. Sauer U, Gittenberger-de Groot AC, Peters DR, Bühlmeyer K (1983) Cineangiocardiography of the coronary arteries in transposition of the great arteries. Ped Cardiol 4 (Suppl):25–42
12. Shaher RM, Puddu GC (1966) Coronary arterial anatomy in complete transposition of the great vessels. Am J Cardiol 17:572–583
13. Viragh SZ, Kalman F, Gittenberger-de Groot AC, Poelmann RE, Moorman AFM (1990) Angiogenesis and hematopoiesis in the epicardium of the vertebrate embryo heart. Ann N Y Acad Sci 588:455–458

Author's address:
A. C. Gittenberger-de Groot
Department of Anatomy
and Embryology
University of Leiden
P.O. Box 9602
2300 RC Leiden
The Netherlands

Transposition of the great arteries: advantages and results of prospective fetal detection. Experience from 1983–1990

L. Fermont
Institute of Puericulture of Paris, France

Introduction

Prenatal cardiology evolved as a speciality after it became feasible to study fetal heart anatomy and function by cross-sectional and Doppler echocardiography. Experience from numerous centers during the last decade indicates that, in experienced hands, this diagnostic method can be as useful, safe, and repeatable as postnatal echocardiography. Prenatal cardiology has developed rapidly and prenatal prospective detection of heart defects is a reality. The real questions in prenatal cardiology today are to define its usefulness, its limitations, and to achieve a maximum of diagnostic accuracy for the benefit of a population new to the pediatric cardiologist: the fetus. Confirmation of fetal heart defects following fetal screening by the obstetrician, counseling of parents with respect to prognosis of the heart defect and possible medical or surgical treatment, and planning of delivery in collaboration with the obstetrician have become tasks of the pediatric cardiologist, who is involved with prenatal cardiology.

The most satisfying aspects of prenatal cardiology involve those heart defects which are grave, but curable, that disturb the fetal circulation and would be potentially fatal if no intrauterine diagnosis and adequate pre- or postnatal treatment were instituted. Transposition of the great arteries represents such a heart defect, and the purpose of this study is to illustrate how prenatal cardiology can be useful for managing the appropriate medical and surgical therapy for the fetus to the centre, which can effect treatment.

General organization of prenatal screening of the heart

Prenatal cardiology is part of fetal medicine and shares its goal to detect fetal anomalies which require adequate neonatal treatment [6]. Examination of the heart by ultrasound should be part of fetal assessment. Obstetricians must be convinced of the potential benefit of detection of fetal heart disease and of the benefits of a program of systematic screening of a population. A cardiac problem is first detected by the obstetrician in the vast majority of cases. The role of the pediatric cardiologist is to confirm the suspected cardiac defect, evaluate its severity with respect to fetal outcome, and assess its effect on postnatal survival with respect to surgical and medical treatment options.

The main responsibility of prenatal cardiology lies with the obstetricians, who are responsible for the conduct of pregnancy, perinatal monitoring, organization of delivery, and detection of fetal pathology among the general population. This can only be achieved if the obstetrician achieves a certain expertise in echocardiography. By training all obstetricians to evaluate the heart in the four-chamber view in all their routine ultrasound fetal examinations many severe heart defects like those associated with hypoplasia of one ventricle, those associated with atresia of an atrioventricular valve, or cardiomyopathies can be detected. By also incorporating the visualization of the origin of the two great vessels into the routine screening program, most conotruncal malformations, transposition, and aortic or pulmonary atresia can be detected.

Prenatal detection of congenital heart disease depends on the activity of obstetricians, which varies from country to country. In France there are at least three fetal ultrasound examinations performed: one early (8–11 weeks of gestation), one intermediate (around 22 weeks of gestation), and one late examination. Most congenital abnormalities including heart defects can be detected at the intermediate examination.

Echocardiographic diagnosis: heart defects in the prenatal period

The echocardiographic examination is conducted in a fashion similar to the postnatal study. An unfavorable fetal position, obesity of the mother, a poor ultrasound abdominal window or paucity of amniotic fluid may interfere with the examination. The segmental approach is used for the echocardiographic examination [1, 4] and the aim is to image the following:

- visceroatrial situs, inferior vena cava, normally to the right of the spine leading to the right atrium. Inferior vena cava flow, well seen by color-coded Doppler is partially deviated to the left atrium via the intraatrial septum. The protrusion of the foramen ovale valve and the direction right-left of the intraatrial shunt indicates the position of the atrial appendage related to caval inflow (usually the right), and of the atrial appendage related to pulmonary vein inflow (usually the left).
- interventricular septum, which divides both ventricles, of which the morphology can be recognized as right or left.
- the two AV valves, which by their morphology and tension apparatus can be identified as tricuspid or mitral valve.
- the ventricular outflow tract and the great vessels: the aorta ascends in a near horizontal caudo-cranial direction and the aortic arch gives rise to head and neck vessels, the pulmonary artery has an oblique direction and normally branches early into a left and right pulmonary artery.

The visceroatrial situs, the intracardiac anatomy, the atrioventricular and ventriculoarterial connections can be identified prenatally [2]. Ventriculoarterial discordance or complete transposition of the great arteries can be diagnosed by the posterior pulmonary artery which originates from the left ventricle and can be identified by its early branching. The aorta is anterior and the direction of the ascending aorta is parallel to the pulmonary artery.

Echocardiography is also capable of analyzing the interventricular septum (intact or with a septal defect of perimenbranous, inlet or outlet type), the aortic arch (normal, with coarctation or interruption), the subpulmonary area (normal or stenosed; with or without deviation of infudibular septum; with or without hypoplasia of pulmonary annulus) and the pulmonary artery.

40

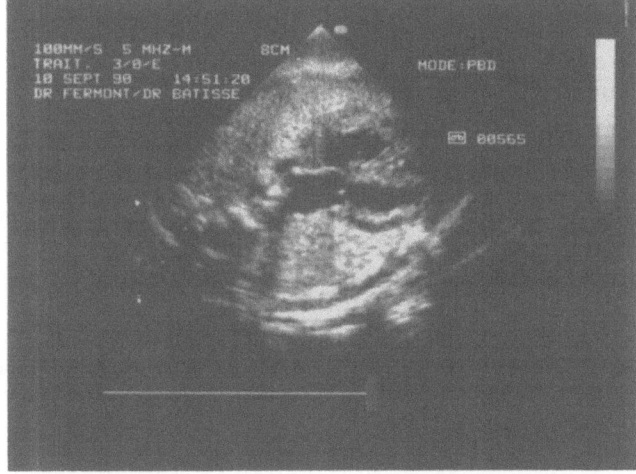

Fig. 1

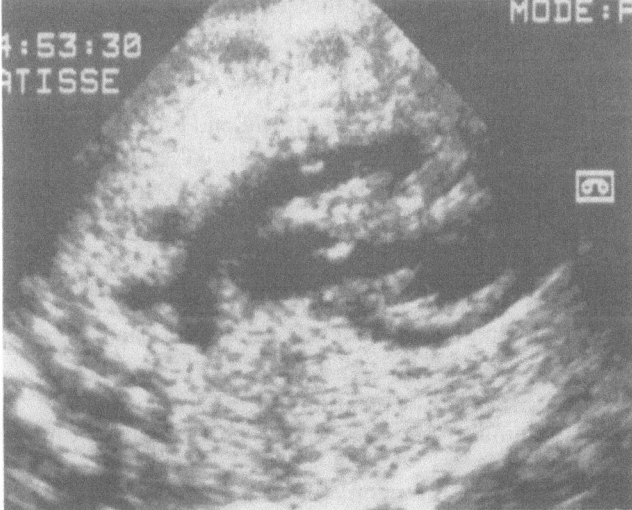

Fig. 2

Fig. 1 and 2. Two dimensional echocardiography in a fetus of 22 weeks gestation: Transposition of the great arteries could be diagnosed, as the vessel leaving the left ventricle could be identified as the pulmonary artery by its branching pattern (Figure 1). Figure 2 confirms that the 2 vessels leaving the heart are parallel with an anterior aorta and a posterior pulmonary artery

Anatomic diagnosis of transposition of the great arteries (Figs. 1 and 2) can readily be made by echocardiography, which is also able to identify additional lesions like ventricular septal defect, coarctation of the aorta or right-ventricular hypoplasia and can exclude other conotruncal malformations like double outlet right ventricle, which, like transposition with ventricular septal defect with or without pulmonary stenosis only rarely puts the neonate at immediate risk.

The addition of color-coded Doppler has made little contribution to improve diagnostic accuracy in isolated transposition of the great vessels. Color-coded Doppler may, however, aid in making statements about the prognosis of transposition, as it helps to better delineate associated defects than two-dimensional echocardiography alone. It may help to identify those complex malformations which constitute neonatal emergencies and can alter the surgical approach, and it also helps parents to better comprehend the nature of the malformations. Color-coded Doppler aids in finding ventricular septal defects in the trabecular part of the interventricular septum, in the study of the conal septum, and the parietal band (if this is deviated anteriorly and impedes subaortic blood flow, one has to fear additional aortic arch obstruction), and in the study of the subpulmonary region. With color-coded Doppler, one can readily and quickly identify turbulent blood flow and the degree of obstruction can subsequently be identified by use of pulsed or continuous wave Doppler. The modified Bernoulli equation can be applied in the fetus in the same way as in the neonate. Normally, blood flow in all great vessels is unidirectional and homogeneous, with a maximal velocity of 1 m/s. In case of an associated coarction of the aorta the flow around the isthmic region is turbulent and of higher velocity at the aortic end of the ductus arteriosus.

The analysis of the pulmonary valve, which may become the aortic valve after the switch operation is important. Minor anatomic abnormalities are frequent and can be detected by the presence of turbulent but often non-stenotic systolic flow or minor localized areas of incompetence. With Doppler, one may also detect a minor tricuspid regurgitation, which is rarely holosystolic and is of little significance if not associated with other fetal pathology.

The study of the foramen ovale is of interest towards the end of the pregnancy, as some fetuses have a prenatal restriction of the foramen ovale. This is especially important to the fetus with transposition as he or she may be in need of an urgent Rashkind balloon septostomy right after delivery.

Possible consequences of prenatal detection

Echocardiographic and Doppler evaluation of the fetal heart is possible. If expertly performed, it allows:

- confirmation of diagnosis of complete transposition of the great arteries
- exclusion of complex associated malformations: single ventricle, atrioventricular septal defect.
- recognition of cases, which may become neonatal emergencies: transposition with intact septum, transposition with coarctation of the aorta, transposition with ventricular septal defect and aortic arch obstruction, restriction of foramen ovale valve.
- distinguishing those cases from pulmonary atresia.
- prenatal planning of type and timing of corrective surgery: early after birth for transposition with intact septum, after a few weeks for transposition with ventricular septal defect, and after some months or years for transposition with pulmonary stenosis.

In most cases, the diagnosis "transposition of the great arteries" is not associated with a chromosomal abnormality or with malformations in other organ systems. Karyotyping the fetus may, nevertheless, be indicated to exclude chromosomal abnormalities in those cases which will almost certainly undergo neonatal cardiac surgery. It is important to confirm that the sole anomaly is the cardiac defect, which is potentially curable and should not lead to termination of pregnancy.

Diagnosis of a heart defect is an indication for repeated fetal ultrasound examinations with emphasis on trying to exclude extracardiac anomalies. It is also important for the psychological guidance of the family, which should be motivated to continue the pregnancy and should be told in detail about the therapeutic options. In general, transposition of the great arteries does not alter the natural course of a pregnancy. The delivery can be vaginal and cesarean section is usually not indicated. The potential request for termination of pregnancy should be refused in view of the current surgical results of treatment of transposition. Rather, the prenatal detection of transposition should lead to a delivery scheduled near a center specialized in pediatric cardiology, where an immediate treatment by Rashkind balloon septostomy can be initiated, if needed. Also, such a center will be able to give prostaglandins in cases with aortic arch abnormalities or pulmonary atresia. Use of prostaglandins should be discouraged in cases of simple transposition without prior echocardiographic confirmation of a nonrestrictive foramen ovale valve in order to avoid potential pulmonary edema.

Prenatal diagnosis of transposition also raises the question of a very early arterial switch operation immediately after birth, without preceding atrial septostomy. This may become possible, theoretically, if surgeons are informed weeks before the delivery and can arrange for surgical repair around the date of delivery. The advantage of this approach over an approach of some days of observation under palliative therapy with balloon septostomy and prostaglandines with or without artificial ventilation has not yet been established. Before this can be done, one should compare morbidity and mortality of neonates who underwent prenatal diagnosis with postnatal echocardiographic confirmation of transposition and then early repair without Rashkind balloon septostomy to the morbidity of Rashkind balloon septostomy. Similarly, one could compare a group of neonates who underwent surgical treatment based on echocardiographic diagnosis alone, to a group who underwent cardiac catheterization with coronary angiography prior to surgery.

Incidence of prenatally detected heart defects

Between January 1983 and December 1990, 5405 women between the ages of 15 and 41 years were seen at our institution for an echocardiographic examination of the fetal heart between the 14th and 41st week of pregnancy. The indications for consulting a pediatric cardiologist could be divided into 2 groups: The group of fetuses at risk and the group seen for expertise. The latter group consisted of fetuses seen after obstetricial screening had revealed suspicion of a cardiac defect, or proper imaging of the heart and/or obtaining the usual views had been difficult.

The risk group included the following patients:
1) antecedents with congenital heart disease, 2) fetal dysrhythmias, 3) ultrasound detection of an extracardiac anomaly, 4) fetal growth-retardation, 5) functional fetal abnormalities like abnormal Doppler in extracardiac vessels or presence of effusions or hydrops, 6) maternal pathology either general disease (diabetes or lupus) or treatment with teratogenic drugs (antiepileptic drugs or lithium) or maternal alcohol abuse.

Overall, 819 congenital heart defects could be detected. The majority of the defects were severe, especially in those coming from the expertise group. In Table 1 we have illustrated that 35.7% of cases in whom a heart defect was suspected by

Table 1. Fetal heart screening. "Non familial" indications

Indications for cardiac screening	Number	CHD detected	%
Total	3286	754	22,9
Maternal diseases and dysfunctions	341	49	14.3
Arrythmias	893	46	5.1
Extra-cardiac defects	314	38	12.1
"2nd-level" study (obstetric screening)	1738	621	35.7

CHD = congenital heart disease

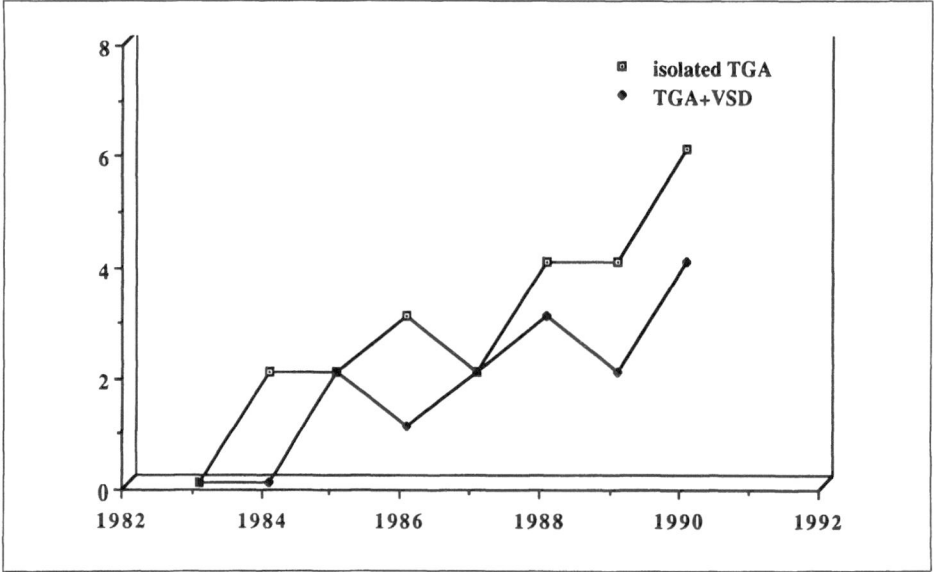

Fig. 3. The annual increase in the number of prenatally detected cases of transposition with or without VSD is shown

obstetricians (with a widely different spectrum of knowledge of congenital heart malformations) had a heart defect. The simple transpositions of the great vessels, the transpositions with coarctation of the aorta, those with ventricular septal defects, and those with a combination of both are potential neonatal emergencies which cannot be diagnosed prospectively unless the systematic evaluation of the origin of the great vessels is added to the four-chamber view examination of the heart. Thus, 92% of the transpositions come from the expertise group of fetal examinations.

The number of detected cardiac malformations has considerably varied over the course of time. As illustrated in Fig. 3, there has been a steady rise of the number of prenatally detected transpositions to 10 cases in 1990, among them six with intact ventricular septum and 4 cases with ventricular septal defect. One each among those groups had associated coarctation of the aorta.

We have observed one case of simple transposition with subsequent familial recurrence in a more complex form associated with mitral atresia and absence of ventricular septum. We have also seen one family with recurrence of double outlet right ventricle. Overall, recurrences in cases of conotruncal malformations are rare in our experience.

The fetal karyotype was studied in all cases by amnio- (n = 7) or chordocentesis (n = 26). We encountered one case of simple transposition with a chromosomal anomaly (deletion of the short arm of chromosome 18) discovered during systematic karyotyping. In contrast to the observations in double outlet ventricle, the association of chromosomal abnormalities with transposition is rare.

Timing of prenatal diagnosis

The mean duration of pregnancy at time of prenatal detection of transposition was 29 weeks; it has been reduced to 26.5 weeks during the last year. Essentially, the diagnosis is made in the third trimester of pregnancy. Only three cases could be detected before 23 weeks of gestation, the earliest case among those, at 19 weeks of gestation, had a complex transposition and mitral atresia and had an older sibling with a simple transposition. Earlier detection could be achived by earlier visualization of the heart with the aid of transvaginal echocardiography. By this technique transposition can be detected as early as 15 weeks of gestation. However, earlier detection has no implications for the diagnosis and management of transposition of the great arteries. But there is a risk of earlier fetal detection in that it may lead a certain number of parents, who are not prepared to accept a „malformed" child, despite expert counseling, to termination of pregnancy. This was case in one of our fetuses in whom detection was achieved at 23 weeks of gestation and in whom termination of pregnancy was performed without our control and against our advice in a "non-official" obstetric unit.

The impact of prenatal detection on outcome in patients with transposition

Among the 819 heart defects, 108 (14.5%) malpositions of the great arteries were detected. Table 2 represents the anatomic diagnosis in more detail. There were 34 transpositions either isolated or with one interventricular septal defect or with coarctation of the aorta. Table 2 also shows that, in contrast to double-outlet right ventricle, chromosomal abnormalities and extracardiac malformations are rarely found in transposition. This partially explains why the number of terminations of pregnancy and medical advice after parental request for termination differ markedly between these two groups. We did not accept any request for termination in the group of simple transposition. The only termination in our experience happened after a strong parental request in a „non-official" obstetrical unit. The other pregnancies were continued even in the case of an antecedent with heart defect and in the one case with chromosomal abnormality. Three terminations were accepted on medical grounds in the group of transposition with ventricular septal defect among them, two because of extracardiac anomalies (one cerebral anomaly and one of the digestive tract) and one (transposition with multiple ventricular septal defects and juxtaposed atrial appendages) because of psychological burden on the

Table 2. Anatomical details and outcome in 108 cases of malposition (DORV, TGA)

Neonatal surgery	Total	Genetic anomalies	Extracardiac malformation	Termination	Fetal death
DORV	16	1	2	7	0
DORV + PS	2	1	0	1	0
DORV + Patr	8	0	0	5	0
DORV + CAVC	12	4	2	6	2
DORV + CAVC + PS	7	3	1	3	1
DORV + CACV + Patr	13	1	2	9	0
	58	10	7	31	3
simple TGA	21	1	0	1	0
simple TGA + Coa	1	0	0	0	0
TGA + VSD	10	0	0	0	0
TGA + VSD + Coa	2	0	0	0	0
TGA + multiple VSD	1	0	0	0	0
TGA + CAVC	1	0	0	1	
TGA + mult VSD + atr. appendage juxtap.	1	0		1	
	37	1	0	3	0
TGA + VSD + PS	9	0	1	1	0
TGA + VSD + Patr	4	0	1	3	0
	13		2	4	
Total	108	11	9	38	3

DORV = double outlet right ventricle, PS = pulmonary stenosis, CAVC = common atrioventricular canal, Patr = pulmonary atresia, Coa = coarcatation of the aorta, VSD = ventricular septal defect, TGA = transposition of the great arteries

mother, which emerged when diagnostic and prognostic uncertainties became apparent. In particular, in the presence of juxtaposed atrial appendages it was difficult to rule out associated ano malous pulmonary venous drainage or atrioventricular septal defect, and multiple examinations by different pediatric cardiologists became necessary before the correct diagnosis could be established.

All prenatal diagnoses were confirmed by neonatal echocardiographic examinations and cardiac catheterization with angiography, and all underwent a Rashkind balloon septostomy.

The mean age of arrival at a specialized cardiac center of a neonate in whom transposition had been detected prenatally was 4.2 h as compared to 14.5 hours in the neonates who had not benefited from prenatal diagnosis. Apart from the terminations, we lost two patients in the neonatal period. One case had been detected at 23 weeks of gestation and died at arrival in a cardiac center from severe acidosis, which could not be reversed despite attempted Rashkind balloon septostomy. The other newborn died from necrotizing enterocolitis after the Rashkind balloon septostomy.

Thirty of the neonates with transposition were surgically treated. Among those four underwent a Senning procedure between 1983 and 1986 at a mean age of 2.7

months. Twenty-six underwent an arterial switch operation at a mean age of 6.3 days for the simple transpositions, at a mean age of 2.4 days in the cases with associated coarctation, and at a mean age of 3.7 weeks in the cases with associated ventricular septal defect. There was no surgical death. One neonate with simple transposition is severely ill as he suffers from pulmonary hypertension which was detected 3 months after the arterial switch operation. He currently is on the waiting list for a heart-lung transplantation.

The overall mortality in this group is 9%, including the case of termination of pregnancy. All cases died before surgical intervention. The mortality could be reduced by reaching a consensus to absolutely refuse termination of pregnancy, which is our policy in cases of transposition, and by improving the coordination between pre- and postnatal care.

Sensitivity and specificity of prenatal diagnosis

During the 7-year period, we encountered two false negatives. Both were seen near term for the first time, when the fetal examination was technically difficult. This should not be an excuse, but it illustrates that the pediatric cardiologist working in fetal medicine should be constantly alert and that the diagnostic chain should not be interrupted: the neonatologist should remain critical and not be prejudiced by the prenatal diagnosis in his assessment of the newborn infant, and he must keep in mind that there may have been a potential error in the fetal diagnosis. Both neonates were immediately correctly diagnosed after birth by the attending neonatalologist and underwent Rashkind balloon septostomy, and later underwent surgical treatment (one Senning in 1983 and one arterial switch in 1988) with excellent results.

We had no false positives in this series except for one case where the suspected diagnosis of transposition with ventricular septal defect was changed in the postnatal examination to corrected transposition with ventricular septal defect and pulmonary stenosis. This error is important in view of the inadequate advice given to parents regarding surgical treatment options and prognosis and the psychological problems which subsequently arose. In effect, this infant, who was born in 1985, has not yet required surgical intervention.

In the future a greater experience may reduce the incidence of diagnostic errors.

Conclusions

This study on prenatal detection of transposition of the great arteries demonstrates that fetal cardiology is an integral part of pediatric cardiology [5] and it requires different technology, obligation of multidisciplinary collaboration, and confrontation with and discussion of ethical issues. The decision to continue a pregnancy in cases of congenital heart defects requires parental guidance, discussion of modification of course of pregnancy with the obstetrician, planning of delivery near a pediatric cardiac center, and prenatal briefing of the neonatologists and cardiac surgeons who will be involved in the treatment of the neonate; only then can the fetus maximally benefit from prenatal detection of the congenital heart defect.

References

1. Allan LD (1986) Manual of fetal echocardiography. Lancaster, MTP Press Ltd.
2. Allan LD, Crawford DC, Chita SK, Tynan MJ (1986) Prenatal screening for congenital heart disease. Br Med J 292:1717–1719
3. Arbeille P, Asquier E, Moxhon E, Magnin M, Pourcelot L, Lansac J (1983) L'étude de la circulation foetale et placentaire par ultrasons. J Gyn Obstet Biol Reprod (Paris) 12:851–859
4. Copel JA, Pilu G, Green J, Hobbins JC, Kleinman CS (1987) Fetal echocardiographic screening for congenital heart disease: the importance of the four-chamber view. Am J Obstet Gynecol 157:648–655
5. Fermont L (1987) Recherche, identification, pronostic et traitement des troubles du rythme et de la conduction chez le foetus. In: Kachaner J, Batisse A (eds) Troubles du rythme cardiaque chez l'enfant. Paris, Doin, pp 37–54
6. Fermont L, Kachaner J, Sidi D (1991) Fetal detection of congenital heart diseases: why and how to screen a population. In: Chervenak FA, Isaacson G, Campbell S (eds) Textbook of Ultrasound in Obstetrics and Gynecology. Boston, Little Brown & Co. (in press)
7. Shenker L, Reed KL, Marx GR, Donnerstein RL, Allen HD, Anderson CF (1988) Fetal Doppler flow studies in prenatal diagnosis of heart diseases. Am J Obstet Gynecol 158:126–173
8. Huhta JC, Strasburger JF, Carpenter RJ, et al. (1985) Pulsed Doppler fetal echocardiography. JCU 13:247–254

Author's address:
Dr. Laurent Fermont
Institut de Puericulture de Paris
26 Boulevard Brune
F-75014 Paris
France

The perinatal circulation and aortopulmonary transposition

A. M. Rudolph
University of California, San Francisco, USA

Major adjustments of the circulation occur after birth. During fetal life, oxygenation is carried out in the placenta, and oxygenated blood returning to the fetal body via the umbilical veins is partly mixed with systemic venous blood. This mixture is then distributed to both the fetal body and the placenta; the fetus has therefore been said to have a circulation in parallel. Following birth, the placental circulation is eliminated and the function of gas exchange is transferred to the lungs, necessitating a marked increase in pulmonary blood flow to supply adequate oxygen to the newborn. In this presentation, the normal fetal circulation is described, and the hemodynamics of the circulation in the presence of transposition of the aorta and pulmonary artery are conjectured. The normal adjustments after birth are then presented, and the interrelationships between postnatal adjustments and aortopulmonary transposition are considered.

Normal fetal circulation

The most detailed description of the course of the fetal circulation has been derived from studies in fetal lambs (Fig. 1). Only recently, since the introduction of ultrasound and Doppler flow studies, has information about the human fetal circulation begun to become available. The circulation in the lamb fetus will be presented, and comparative information in the human fetus considered.

Oxygenated blood returns to the fetus from the placenta through the umbilical vein, which enters the porta hepatis. About half the umbilical venous blood is distributed to the liver; the remainder passes through the ductus venosus to the inferior vena cava. Ductus venosus blood, with the high oxygen saturation of umbilical venous blood, preferentially streams in the inferior vena cava to pass across the foramen ovale to the left atrium. Systemic venous blood from the abdominal inferior vena cava preferentially streams across the tricuspid valve into the right ventricle. Because of this selective streaming of superior vena caval blood and the preferential streaming of ductus venosus and abdominal inferior vena caval blood, the oxygen saturation of blood in the right ventricle is about 50%, whereas that in the left atrium and left ventricle is about 65%.

In the fetal lamb, the right ventricle ejects about 65% of the total combined output of the heart, and the left ventricle ejects about 35% of combined ventricular output (CVO). CVO is about 450 mL/min/kg fetal body weight. The right ventricle ejects into the pulmonary trunk; most of the right ventricular output is directed through the ductus arteriosus into the descending aorta (55% of CVO). Only 8–10% of CVO passes through the pulmonary circulation. Left-ventricular blood is ejected into the aorta to supply blood with a relatively high oxygen saturation of

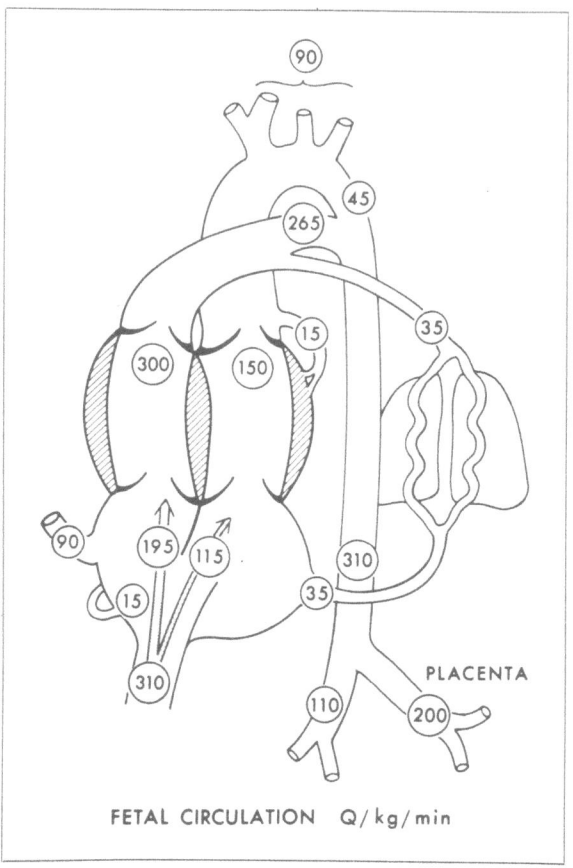

Fig. 1. The course of the circulation in the normal fetus. Numbers in circles represent the volumes of blood (per kg fetal weight) flowing through the cardiac chambers and great vessels in the lamb

about 65% to the coronary circulation (3% CVO), head, brain, and forelimbs (about 20% CVO). The remaining 8–10% of left-ventricular blood passes across the aortic isthmus to the descending aorta to join the blood entering from the ductus arteriosus. Descending aortic blood, with an oxygen saturation of about 55%, constitutes about 70% of CVO. Forty percent of CVO is distributed to the umbilical-placental circulation, and the remaining 30% supplies the abdominal organs, lower trunk, and hindlimbs (Fig. 1).

In the human fetus, Doppler flow studies have shown that the general flow patterns described in the lamb are similar. However, because the body configurations are different, the proportions of CVO distributed to the upper and lower body are not the same. The most important difference is in the brain size, particularly because the brain has a high blood flow per unit weight of tissue. The human fetal brain constitutes about 13% of body weight, while the sheep brain is only 2–3% of body weight. If it is assumed that blood flow per unit weight of brain is similar in the

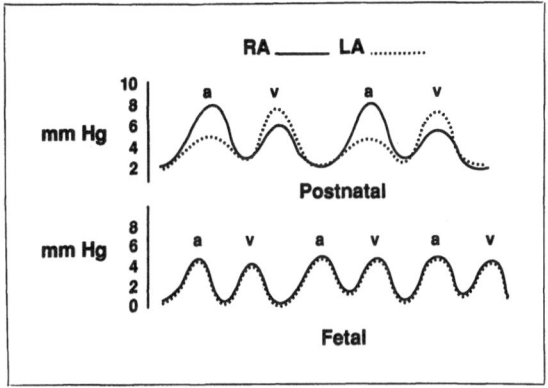

Fig. 2. Atrial pressure contours during the fetal and postnatal periods are diagrammatically presented. In the fetus, normally, right and left atrial pressures are similar throughout the cardiac cycle. Postnatally, the left atrial "v" wave becomes dominant as a result of increased pulmonary blood flow. Right atrial pressure shows a dominant "a" wave

sheep and human fetus, the volume of blood necessary for the left ventricle to supply the additional flow to the brain can be calculated. Based on these assumptions, the left and right ventricular outputs would be similar in the human fetus. Echocardiographic studies in the human fetus have confirmed this, showing that the estimated ratio of right:left ventricular output is about 1.2−1.3 : 1.0 as compared with the lamb fetus, in which it is 2 : 1.

In the lamb fetus, blood entering the left ventricle consists of the 8−10% CVO returning from the lungs and about 25% of CVO that passes through the foramen ovale from the inferior vena cava. In the human fetus, the left ventricle ejects almost 50% of CVO; whether the additional volume is derived from a relatively larger pulmonary blood flow, or whether it is from flow through the foramen ovale, is yet to be determined.

Pressures in the cardiac chambers and great vessels are greatly influenced by the fetal shunts. The foramen ovale provides a large communication between the inferior vena cava and left atrium. Pressure in the venae cavae and right atrium is consistently higher than left atrial pressure throughout the whole cardiac cycle, with constant flow from the inferior vena cava and right atrium to the left atrium (Fig. 2). The phasic contours of the pressures in the right and left atria are almost identical, with a larger "a" than "v" wave. Systolic pressures in the left and right ventricles are almost similar, but end-diastolic pressure is about 1 mmHg higher in the right ventricle. The ductus arteriosus is a large connection between the pulmonary trunk and descending aorta, and thus both systolic and diastolic pressures in the aorta and pulmonary arteries are similar. Because pulmonary vascular resistance is very high in the fetus, blood flows from the pulmonary trunk through the ductus arteriosus throughout the cardiac cycle. Flow is directed almost entirely into the descending aorta, because vascular resistance in the distribution of the ascending aorta is much higher than that in the distribution of the descending aorta, which includes the relatively low-resistance placental circulation.

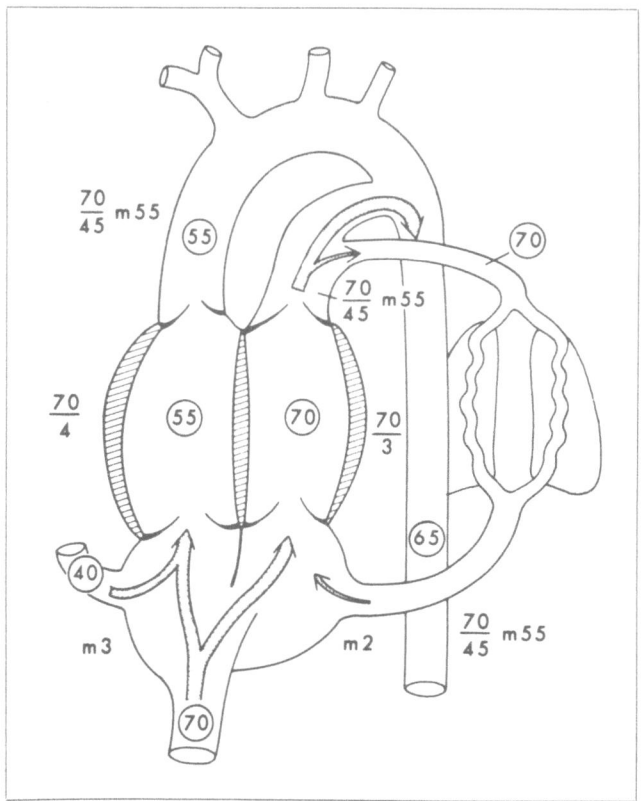

Fig. 3. The course of fetal circulation in the presence of aortopulmonary transposition. Based on these flow patterns, it is hypothesized that pulmonary arterial oxygen saturation is higher than in the normal fetus, and that ascending aortic oxygen saturation would be lower. Also, unlike in the normal fetus, descending aortic oxygen saturation would be higher than in the ascending aorta

Fetal hemodynamics and aortopulmonary transposition

The presence of shunts through the foramen ovale and ductus arteriosus in the fetus permits adequate distribution of oxygenated blood to the body, so that transposition should have little impact on normal in utero development. The main effect of transposition would be to alter the normal oxygen saturation difference between blood distributed to the upper and lower parts of the body (Fig. 3). The venous flow patterns would not be influenced greatly by aortopulmonary transposition; the preferential streaming of ductus venosus blood across the foramen ovale would provide blood with higher oxygen saturation to the left atrium and ventricle. The superior vena caval blood with low oxygen saturation, as well as preferentially directed abdominal venous blood would enter the right ventricle. However, the right ventricular blood with lower oxygen saturation would be ejected into the ascending aorta, so that the myocardium and brain would receive blood of somewhat lower oxygen saturation than normal (probably about 50% instead of 65%). This probably would not affect oxygen supply to the myocardium and brain,

52

because oxygen delivery can readily be maintained to these organs, even with severe fetal hypoxemia, by the increased blood flow associated with vasodilation.

Left-ventricular blood, with its higher oxygen saturation of about 65%, would be ejected into the pulmonary trunk and be distributed to the pulmonary circulation, as well as through the ductus arteriosus to the descending aorta. Because the pulmonary circulation is very sensitive to relatively small changes in oxygen tension of blood perfusing the lungs, pulmonary vascular resistance could be lower, and pulmonary blood flow higher than normal. This could reduce the volume of inferior vena caval blood passing through the foramen ovale because of the higher pulmonary venous return to the left atrium. The distribution of blood with a higher than normal oxygen saturation to lower body organs and the placenta probably does not have any significant influence.

Cardiovascular adjustments after birth

Following birth, oxygen supply to the newborn must be derived through the lungs, associated with initiation of ventilation and elimination of the umbilical-placental circulation. In the adult circulation, blood flows serially from the left ventricle through the aorta and systemic circulation, then back to the heart through the venae cavaeto the right atrium and ventricle, to be ejected through the pulmonary circulation, returning then to the left atrium and ventricle. To establish this circulation, all fetal shunt pathways must be closed. Studies we have conducted in lambs, either ventilated in utero or delivered by cesarean section, have delineated many of the cardiovascular changes and the mechanisms responsible.

We have shown that the most important event occurring at birth that is responsible for reorientation of the circulation is the fall in pulmonary vascular resistance associated with ventilation. During fetal life, the high pulmonary vascular resistance is maintained by constriction of the well-developed smooth muscle in the pulmonary arterioles. Ventilation with air results in an immediate fall in pulmonary vascular resistance, with and eight- to 10-fold increase in pulmonary blood flow. Two separate mechanisms appear to be responsible for this change. Rhythmic physical expansion of the lung, with no change in oxygen or carbon dioxide concentrations in blood, results in a major fall in pulmonary vascular resistance (Fig. 4). This appears to be related to release of a prostaglandin, probably prostacyclin, because it is inhibited by administration of a prostaglandin synthesis inhibitor such as indomethacin prior to ventilation. The other factor reducing pulmonary vascular resistance is oxygen; this appears to exert its action by releasing endothelial-derived relaxing factor (EDRF), which is a potent vasodilator of the pulmonary vessels.

The dramatic fall in pulmonary vascular resistance, associated with the increased pulmonary flow, results in almost complete elimination of the right-to-left shunt of blood through the ductus arteriosus from the pulmonary trunk to the aorta; while the ductus is still open, a small left-to-right shunt develops. With the increased venous return to the left atrium, the foramen ovale is functionally closed, and the flow of blood from right to left is curtailed. All these changes occur even if the umbilical-placental circulation is left intact. Elimination of the placental circulation by clamping or cutting the umbilical cord reduces venous return via the ductus venosus and inferior vena cava, and results in an elevation of aortic pressure.

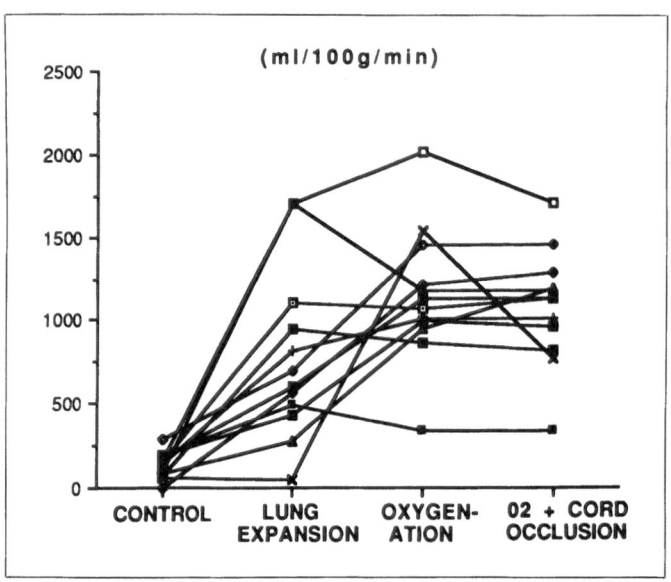

Fig. 4. Changes in pulmonary blood flow associated with birth events in fetal lambs in utero. Ventilating the lamb with a gas that does not change fetal blood gases results in a marked increase in flow in many animals. Ventilating with oxygen produces an additional increase in flow in most of the lambs. Umbilical cord occlusion had no additional effect

The fall in pulmonary vascular resistance is associated with a drop of pulmonary arterial diastolic and mean pressures, but while the ductus arteriosus is widely patent, systolic pressure falls only slightly. Pulmonary arterial pressure falls to near low adult levels when the ductus arteriosus closes. Associated with increased pulmonary venous return and closure of the foramen ovale, left atrial pressure increases above that in the right atrium. There is also a change in the left atrial pressure contour, with the development of a dominant "v" wave, as compared with the right atrium, which retains its dominant "a" wave (Fig. 2).

Ventilation with air results in an increase of arterial oxygen saturation to close to 100% within a short period after birth, and saturation of blood in the ascending and descending aorta is the same. Following these changes that occur within minutes after birth, further adaptations occur. The ductus arteriosus gradually closes; closure is usually complete by 10–15 h after birth. This closure is partly related to the increase in PO_2 of blood to which the ductus arteriosus is exposed. During fetal life it is exposed to the PO_2 of pulmonary arterial blood, about 18 torr, whereas after birth it is exposed to the PO_2 of aortic blood, which soon reaches 90 torr or more. It is also partly related to a reduction in circulating levels of prostaglandin (PGE_2), which helps to maintain ductus patency in the fetus. Changes in other vasoactive agents may be involved. Over the weeks following birth, further changes occur in the pulmonary circulation. Closure of the ductus arteriosus completes the separation of the left and right sides of the heart, and pulmonary arterial pressures fall further. The pulmonary vascular smooth muscle layer becomes thinner over the weeks following birth, resulting in a further fall in pulmonary vascular resistance to the low levels encountered in the adult.

Postnatal circulatory adjustment with aortopulmonary transposition

When the fetus is separated from the umbilical-placental circulation after birth, oxygen must be supplied by the lungs through the pulmonary circulation. With transposition, the pulmonary artery arises from the left ventricle, so that oxygenated blood returning from the lungs is recirculated into the pulmonary circulation. Also systemic venous blood returns to the right atrium and right ventricle, to be ejected into the aorta and recirculated to systemic circulation. For the infant to survive after birth, systemic venous blood must be passed through the lungs to be oxygenated, and pulmonary venous blood must enter the systemic circulation to provide oxygen to the body. This can be accomplished only if shunts between the systemic and pulmonary circulations, in both directions, can be achieved. Following birth, the fetal shunting sites at the foramen ovale and ductus arteriosus levels are capable of providing shunts under certain circumstances. Also presence of a ventricular septal defect may provide another site for shunting. In this presentation, I will discuss the hemodynamics in aortopulmonary transposition in the absence of a ventricular septal defect, or in the presence of only a small ventricular septal defect, because it is usually these patients who present with symptoms in the early neonatal period. Because a large ventricular defect supplies a site for considerable shunting, oxygenation of systemic arterial blood is usually manifest some weeks after birth, rather than in the first few days, as occurs with intact ventricular septum.

Role of the ductus arteriosus

In infants with aortopulmonary transposition, the ductus arteriosus is often patent for a longer period after birth than normal. This could be related to the fact that the ductus continues to be exposed to a relatively low oxygen content derived from the aorta, when pulmonary vascular resistance has fallen, with a resultant flow from the aorta to the pulmonary artery. While the ductus arteriosus is still widely patent and pulmonary resistance has not dropped to very low levels, pulmonary arterial pressure is maintained at relatively high levels, and shunting may occur in a bidirectional manner. During systole, the velocity of blood ejected by the left ventricle into the pulmonary artery carries it through the ductus arteriosus to the descending aorta. During diastole, because pulmonary vascular resistance is lower than that in the systemic circulation, blood flows from the aorta to the pulmonary artery and into the lung circulation. This bidirectional shunt is well visualized either by angiography or by Doppler velocity studies, and the magnitude may be large enough to permit adequate oxygenation of the infant. Because well oxygenated blood from the pulmonary artery is distributed through the ductus arteriosus to the descending, the oxygen saturation may be higher in descending than in ascending aortic blood.

If pulmonary vascular resistance remains high, as, for example, when pulmonary ventilation is inadequate or pulmonary disease or atelectasis is present, shunting through the ductus arteriosus will occur only from the pulmonary artery to the aorta, resulting in a wider separation of oxygen saturations in the ascending and descending aorta. If, however, pulmonary vascular resistance falls markedly and the ductus arteriosus constricts, but is still patent, pulmonary arterial systolic and diastolic pressures will fall, and only aortic-to-pulmonary-arterial shunting will occur. This shunting into the pulmonary circulation may result in pulmonary edema, depending on the behavior of the foramen ovale (see below).

The importance of the ductus arteriosus in maintaining bidirectional shunting in the early postnatal period explains the value of infusion of prostaglandin E_1 in infants with transposition. The use of PGE_1 to dilate the ductus when it is beginning to constrict is often very effective in improving oxygenation in these infants.

Role of the foramen ovale

The foramen ovale may permit postnatal survival of the infant with aortopulmonary transposition by allowing either bidirectional shunting or unidirectional shunting from the right to the left atrium. Bidirectional shunting results when there is an adequate communication between the two atria during all phases of the cardiac cycle, and when the normal postnatal increase in the magnitude of the "v" wave occurs following the increase in pulmonary blood flow. Thus, during atrial systole, shunting through the foramen ovale occurs from the right to left atrium, whereas shunting from the left to right atrium occurs with the "v" wave. The competency of the foramen ovale flap is important in determining the magnitude of left-to-right atrial shunt. If the foramen flap seals the opening completely when left atrial pressure increases, no left-to-right atrial shunting can occur; usually, it leaves a variably sized opening through which there is some shunt. Right-to-left atrial shunting can occur until the foramen is closed anatomically. The Rashkind procedure opens the foramen ovale by tearing the lower flap, thus permitting bidirectional shunting.

Shunting from the systemic to pulmonary circulation is necessary to direct venous blood to the lungs for oxygenation, and from the pulmonary to systemic circulation to provide oxygenated blood to the body tissues. The magnitude of shunt in each direction must be the same; otherwise, there would be a progressive accumulation of blood volume in one circulation and depletion from the other.

If the foramen ovale is competent and the ductus arteriosus is partly constricted, a clinical picture of severe pulmonary edema, unusual with aortopulmonary transposition with intact ventricular septum, can result. With the postnatal fall in pulmonary vascular resistance, pulmonary arterial pressure drops when the ductus arteriosus is partly constricted, and only a shunt from the aorta to the pulmonary artery occurs, resulting in an increase in volume in the pulmonary circuit. Left atrial pressure increases, but with the foramen ovale functionally sealed, no decompression can occur. Progressive increase in pressure results in pulmonary edema. Because shunting from the systemic to pulmonary circulation is restricted, hypoxemia becomes progressively more severe.

Role of pulmonary vascular resistance

The fall in pulmonary vascular resistance is the primary mechanism responsible for the elimination of the right-to-left ductus arteriosus shunt, the increase in pulmonary blood flow, and the closure of the foramen ovale after birth in the normal infant (see above). In infants with aortopulmonary transposition, the pulmonary vascular resistance is of paramount importance in determining the clinical features by influencing shunting patterns. While the ductus arteriosus is still widely open, the fall in pulmonary vascular resistance permits shunting in diastole from the aorta to pulmonary artery. If the pulmonary vascular resistance increases, as with ventilatory disturbance, only pulmonary-arterial-to-aortic shunting occurs. Cyanosis will then be more severe.

The increase in pulmonary blood flow associated with the fall in pulmonary vascular resistance results in the assumption of the dominant "v" wave in the left atrial pressure pulse. If the foramen ovale is incompetent or an atrial septal defect is present, then bidirectional atrial shunting will occur. Following the achievement of a successful tear in the atrial septum with a Rashkind procedure, little improvement in cyanosis may result if the pulmonary vascular resistance is still markedly elevated. Even in the presence of a large atrial communication, the lack of differences in pressure pulse contours between the left and right atria will limit the amount of bidirectional shunt.

In summary, survival of infants with aortopulmonary transposition after birth is possible if fetal shunting sites persist at the ductus arteriosus or foramen ovale, or both. However, the fall in pulmonary vascular resistance is of crucial importance to survival, in addition to persistence of the shunts.

Author's address:
Abraham M. Rudolph, M.D.
Professor of Pediatrics and Obstetrics,
Gynecology & Reproductive Sciences
Neider Professor of Pediatric Cardiology
Senior Staff, Cardiovascular Research Institute
Box 0544, HSE 1403
University of California, San Francisco
San Francisco CA 94143-0544

Balloon atrial septostomy: The Rashkind procedure (1965–1990) – historical and technical aspects

M. H. Paul

Department of Pediatrics, Northwestern University Medical School, Chicago, IL, USA, and Department of Biomedical Engineering, Northwestern University, Evanston, IL, USA

Introduction

This presentation is dedicated to the humanist and physician, William J. Rashkind, and in particular, to his contributions in the development of balloon atrial septostomy as applied to the therapy of transposition of the great arteries.

In a larger sense, however, we celebrate William Rashkind as the *father of interventional cardiac catheterization* – a new discipline now in explosive adolescent bloom – providing astounding new nonsurgical transcatheter treatments for many forms of heart disease in children and adults.

In the 20th century, penetration into the human cardiac chambers by catheter was first performed by Werner Forssmann in 1929 by inserting a ureteral catheter into his own left antecubital vein under fluoroscopic control [7], but it was not until the early 1940s that Andre Cournand and his collaborators initiated the first comprehensive clinical and physiological cardiopulmonary investigative catheterization program [4].

From the fountainhead of Forssmann's bold achievement and the continuing expansion of Cournand's cardiac catheterization methodology there have emerged two derivative catheter-based disciplines. Late in the 1940s and in the 1950s diagnostic, physiologic and selective angiocardiographic studies on congenital heart disease were initiated, and then widely disseminated in the 1960s.

William Rashkind clearly *astounded his colleagues* with a historic 10-min presentation on October 23, 1965, at the Cardiology Section meetings of the American Academy of Pediatrics in Chicago, in describing a therapeutic (palliative) triumph over transposition of the great arteries in three infants using an inflated balloon on a cardiac catheter to create an atrial septal defect (Fig. 1).

The birth of interventional cardiac catheterization

It was thus, in the 1960s that the second derivative of the cardiac catheter, *interventional cardiac catheterization,* was given active life by Rashkind and his collaborators. Rashkind extended this achievement over the next 20 years persistently and brilliantly with development, experimental, and clinical work to fabricate innovative devices and techniques for nonsurgical closure of patent ductus arteriosus and atrial septal defect [14]. A massive expansion of the arena for interventional cardiac catheterization came in 1978 when Andreas Gruentzig reported percutaneous transluminal catheter angioplasty (PTCA) for coronary artery stenosis [9], and later when the balloon catheter became a tool for valvoplasty and large-vessel angioplasty.

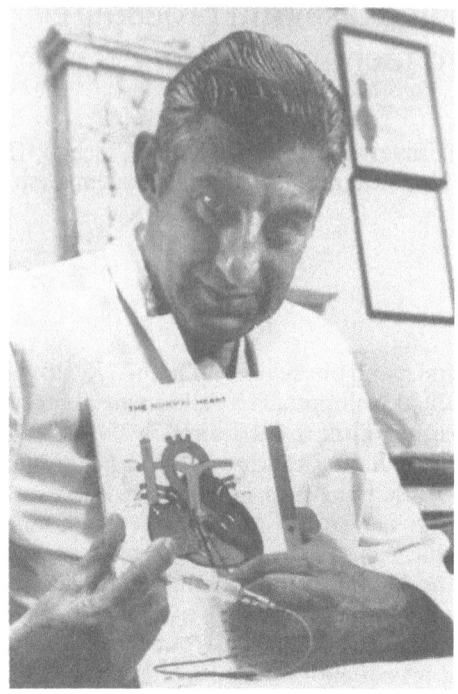

Fig. 1. William J. Rashkind, M.D. (1968) demonstrating balloon catheter. A leading catheter-design engineer (USCI) remembers: "Most of our business was consummated with a handshake; he had the strongest handshake of any man I ever knew! To think that those large hands worked on such tiny bodies!"

So important and pervasive have these new catheter-delivered interventional techniques become (we include catheter-based therapeutic electrophysiologic procedures for "permanently" terminating various tachyarrhythmias) that Alexander Nadas has spoken of the *"chirurgification of cardiology"*. Thus, the image of the cardiologist as the prototype contemplative, wise physician dressed in a white coat and viewing an analog electrocardiogram, chest x-ray or angiocardiogram has been transformed into that of a scrub-suited activist bearing an armamentarium of peculiar catheters with balloons, umbrellas, clamshells, electrodes, and coils. This cardiologist stares intently through radiation protective glasses at digital control panels and imaging screens, as he both diagnoses and *repairs* cardiovascular abnormalities.

Career development

William Rashkind's conceptualization, development, and clinical application of the cardiac catheters as a therapeutic device did not spring forth from an unprepared mind and hand. Following medical studies at the University of Louisville, Kentucky, his interests in formal cardiovascular physiology and physiological measurement techniques engaged him for 6 years (1946–1952) at the Naval Medical Research Institute and the University of Pennsylvania [12], before turning to training in pediatrics and pediatric cardiology at the Children's Hospital of Philadelphia.

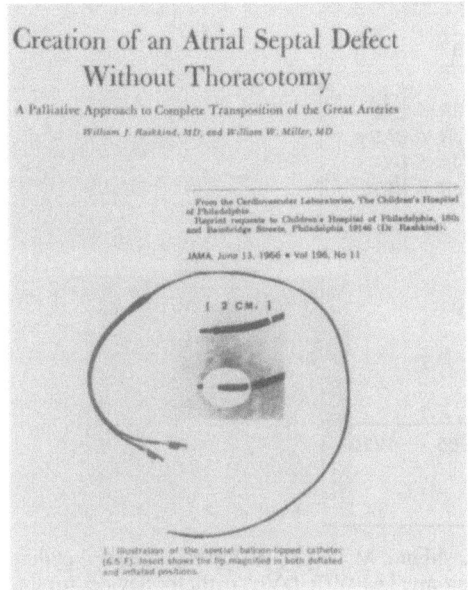

Creation of an Atrial Septal Defect
Without Thoracotomy

A Palliative Approach to Complete Transposition of the Great Arteries

William J. Rashkind, MD, and William W. Miller, MD

Fig. 2. Publication, William J. Rashkind,
M.D. and William W. Miller, M.D., 1966

The Index Contribution

Rashkind's index contribution (Fig. 2) titled, "Creation of an atrial septal defect without thoracotomy: A palliative approach to complete transposition of the great arteries" [15], was published in 1966 with his colleague William W. Miller, 8 years after he was appointed director of the cardiac catheterization laboratory at the Children's Hospital of Philadelphia. There followed, until his death in 1986, a succession of publications (Fig. 3): some eight papers concerned with balloon atrial septostomy [●]; eight papers concerned with various other types of interventional catheter devices [▲]; five unique historical papers on topics relevant to pediatric cardiology [■]; and thirty papers on assorted other pediatric cardiology subjects [○].

The balloon atrial septostomy procedure had immediate worldwide acceptance as the initial treatment for the infant with transposition of the great arteries. There soon followed an outpouring of reports (Fig. 4) that continue even now concerned primarily with clinical assessments [○]; related complications [▲]; umbilical vein approach [■]; and two-dimensional (2-D) echocardiography guidance techniques [■].

Pursuit of an Idea

Several years earlier (1963), in an abstract read at the American Heart Association Scientific Sessions [13], Rashkind reported his experimental efforts to incise the atrial septum with a device (wire and hook) that could be passed through a standard cardiac catheter and presumably replace the "formidable high-risk Blalock-Hanlon and direct vision atrial septum excision surgical procedures for these fragile

61

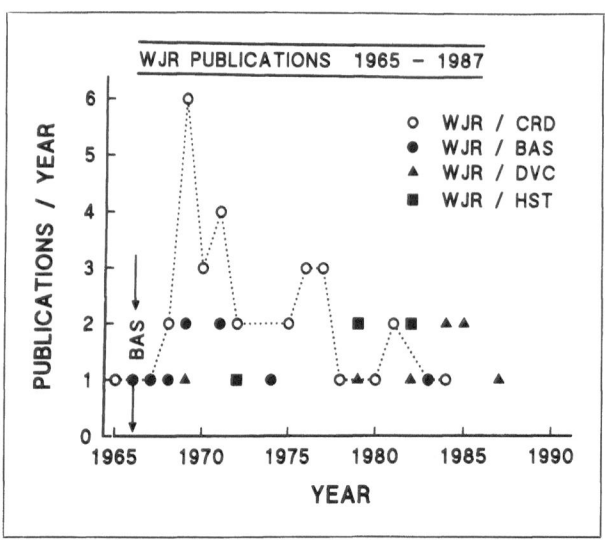

Fig. 3. Publications (1965–1987), William J. Rashkind, M.D. [○] WJR/CRD, general pediatric cardiology; [●] WJR/BAS, balloon atrial septostomy; [▲] WJR/DVC, catheter devices for interventional procedures; [■] WJR/HST, historical reviews

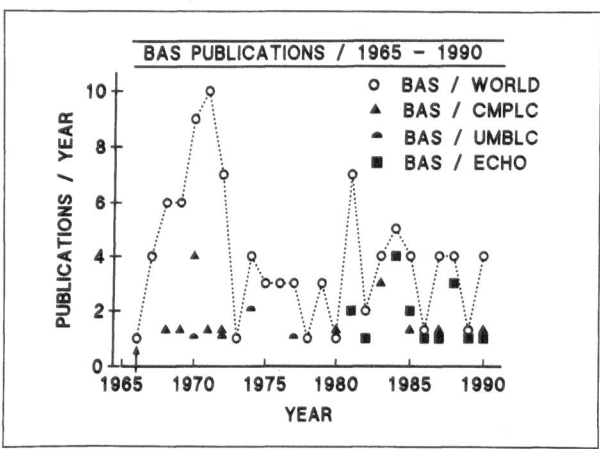

Fig. 4. Publications (1966–1990) concerned with balloon atrial septostomy (BAS) from Medlars listing. [○] BAS, worldwide clinical reports; [▲] BAS/CMPL, complications; [■] BAS/UMBLC, umbilical vein approach; [■] BAS/ECHO, 2-D echocardiography guidance

infants". The wire maneuver was not always successful, and the incision-tears often closed over, and presumably no clinical trials were undertaken.

Rashkind's attention and industry were now directed to the unlikely and audacious concept of rupturing the septum primum flap of the fossa ovalis (Fig. 5) using the force generated by tugging on a semi-rigid fluid-inflated balloon appended to a catheter. *An idea so audaciously simple and creative as to constitute an act of genius!*

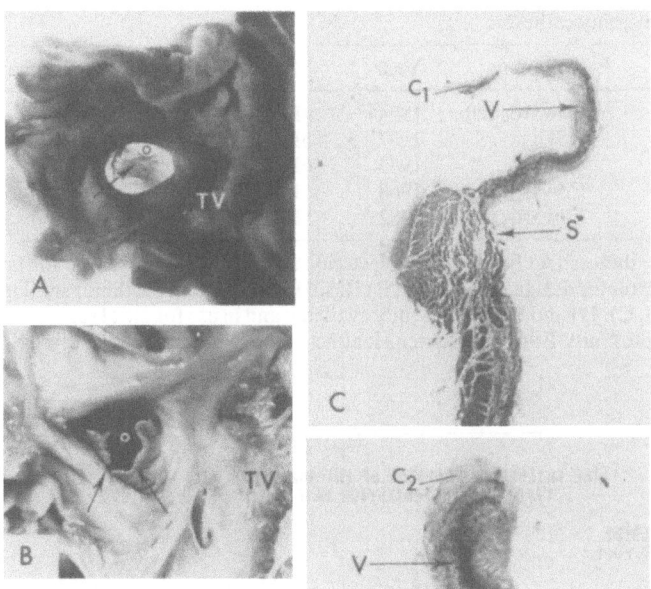

Fig. 5. Fossa ovalis morphology. A) Normal premature infant showing transilluminated right atrial view of thin septum primum valve and elliptical patent foramen ovale (o). B) Infant with transposition of the great arteries showing long, linear tear in septum primum valve at autopsy shortly after septostomy procedure. C) Histologic appearance: C_1, usual thin valve tissue present in most neonates with transposition; and C_2, thick, fibromuscular, balloon-resistant valve tissue encountered in some older infants, particularly with large ventricular septal defect

The concept of surgically creating intercirculatory mixing defects for palliation of transposition had much earlier been discussed by Blalock and Hanlon (1950) – "the duration of life (for an infant with transposition) depends on the degree of mixing between the two circulations" [3], and closed atrial septectomy was being performed, but usually with a significant early surgical risk.

Rashkind's new concept of using a balloon-tipped catheter rather than an incising wire or instrument possibly had several sources of inspiration. First, certainly the world of urological surgery was long populated with numerous catheter interventional devices: instruments such as ureteral stone-extractors and the Foley balloon-bearing bladder drainage catheter. Second, there was the exciting contemporary work of Dotter and Judkins on the use of successively larger dilating catheters to effect nonsurgical transluminal recannulation of obstructed arteriosclerotic vessels in the lower extremity [5].

Third, Rashkind apparently had contact with the recently available (1963) balloon-bearing catheter devised by Fogarty et al. [6] to extract arterial emboli and thrombi. His experimental experience with such a catheter is said to have been unsatisfactory and hence it was abandoned. Of some interest, and discussed later, is the subsequent engineering development program initiated by Paul in 1967 with the Edwards Laboratories to modify the Fogarty arterial embolectomy catheter (Table 1).

Table 1. Balloon atrial septostomy catheters

Design	Company	Year	Shaft/Sheath	Volume/Diameter
A) Fogarty	Edwards Labs	1964	4F/5F	75 ml/9 mm
B) Rashkind	USCI	1967	5F/6F	2.0 ml/14 mm
C) Rashkind (Recessed)	USCI	1982	6F/6F	2.0 ml/14 mm
D) Fogarty (Paul)	Edwards Labs	1968	5F/7F	1.8 ml/15 mm
E) (Fogarty) Miller	Edwards Labs	1982	5F/8,9F	4.0 ml/19 mm

Balloon atrial septostomy catheters: A) Fogarty embolectomy catheter was a prototype for later Edwards Labs septostomy catheter designs D) and E); B) Rashkind septostomy catheter similar to orginal design. Catheters B), C), D) and E) are presently available and in use for atrial septostomy. Company: Edwards Labs, presently Edwards-Baxter Healthcare Corp.; USCI, presently USCI-CR Bard, Inc.

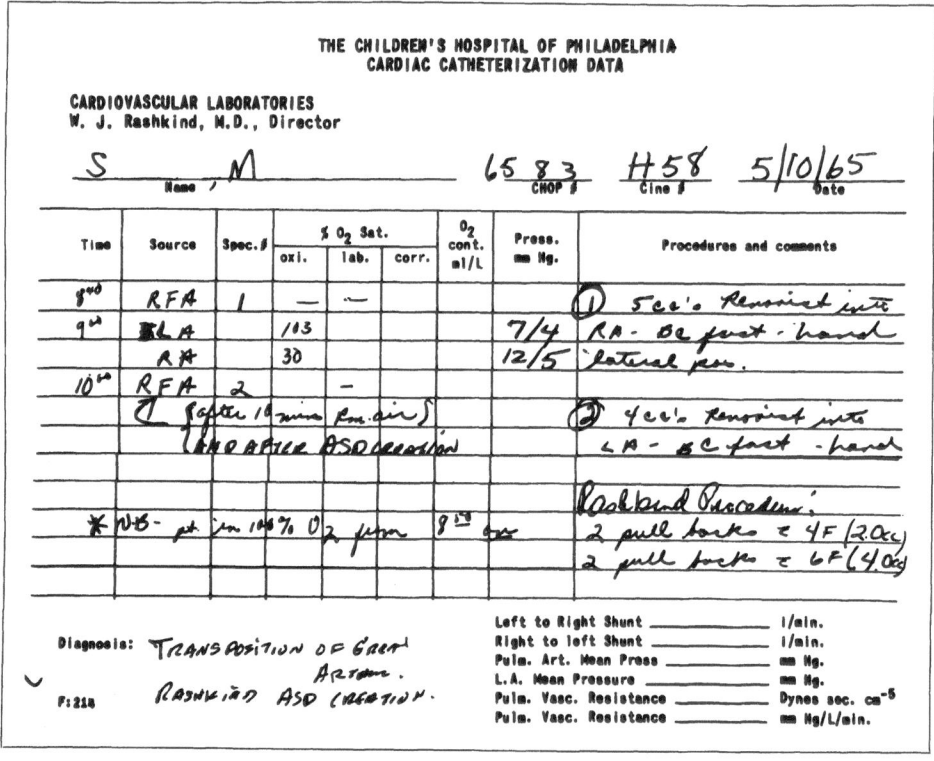

Fig. 6. Catheterization log entries dated may 10, 1965, recording the proceedings of the first clinical balloon atrial septostomy.

In any event, Rashkind, with his associates, set about to fabricate experimental balloon catheters. The first balloons were fashioned on glass rods which had been dipped into liquid latex – a technique he probably had practiced often in the course of experiments in the classical physiology or pharmacology laboratory. Rashkind's personal interest and expertise in tying fishing-flies (lures) provided the means of laboriously mounting the balloon on the distal end of a 6F angiography catheter.

Perhaps Rashkind's philosophy, genius, and tenacity for approaching and solving problems were reflected in the sign he placed prominently in his office and animal laboratory: KISS (an acronym for "Keep It Simple, Stupid")!

Once the efficacy of these crude catheters was proven in newborn puppies, he initiated development of a double lumen septostomy catheter in collaboration with engineers at United States Catheter and Instrument Co., and by 1968 the USCI product catalog included 5.5F, 6.5F double lumen, and 4F, 5F single lumen balloon catheters. The single lumen catheters were considered sufficient for safe localization within the left atrium in conjunction with biplane fluoroscopy, which was becoming readily available. In 1982, USCI/Bard introduced an improved 6F recessed (low-profile) balloon catheter (Table 1).

Quite possibly, the KISS principle is also reflected in the terse catheterization record of may 10, 1965 which describes the first clinical application of the atrial septostomy catheter (Fig. 6): "Rashkind procedure: 2 pull backs c̄ 4F (2.0cc) and 2 pull backs c̄ 6F (4.0cc)."

Twenty-six years later this patient is alive and well, although she sustained a cerebral vascular accident in the interval between septostomy and Mustard atrial repair at 3 years of age. Another apocryphal KISS incident is related by a technician eyewitness who once timed Rashkind in the cath lab in the middle of the night; "58 seconds from touch of knife on skin to balloon in the left atrium!"

In summary, the astounding result of this work was that Rashkind's balloon atrial septostomy, teamed appropriately with a Senning or Mustard atrial repair, progressively *transformed the probability of survival* for the fragile, intensively hypoxemic neonate with complete transposition and intact ventricular septum from less than 10% to 90% or better.

The Edwards Laboratories (Baxter) Fogarty atrial dilation catheter

Dr. Rashkind's announcement, on October 23, 1965, in Chicago, describing successful balloon atrial septostomy coincided with the admission of a newborn with transposition of the great arteries to our cardiology service at the Children's Memorial Hospital, Chicago. Since the newly developed USCI balloon catheter (Fig. 7, R) was not readily available, we obtained a 4F Fogarty embolectomy catheter (Fig. 7, F) from a peripheral vascular surgeon and effected a satisfactory physiologic and clinical response with a 9-mm diameter distended balloon.

Although this first patient in our septostomy experience also went on to have a Mustard atrial repair at 3 years of age, and survived some 25 years after the septostomy procedure, there were increasingly frequent episodes of atrial flutter/tachycardia and, eventually, severe right-ventricular dysfunction. Cardiac transplantation was successful, but severe, sudden rejection resulted in death 1 year later in 1990.

This first septostomy experience in November 1965 caused us to initiate a collaborative program with Edwards Laboratories which resulted in an atrial septostomy catheter based on the Fogarty embolectomy catheter (Fig. 7, F), but with special advanced design features including: 1) a fixed 30°-tip angulation which facilitated manipulation through the foramen ovale; 2) a heavy-walled balloon with controlled-symmetrical balloon geometry mounted over a wire-wound catheter body; 3) a balloon mounting such that the inflated medium passes to and from the balloon

65

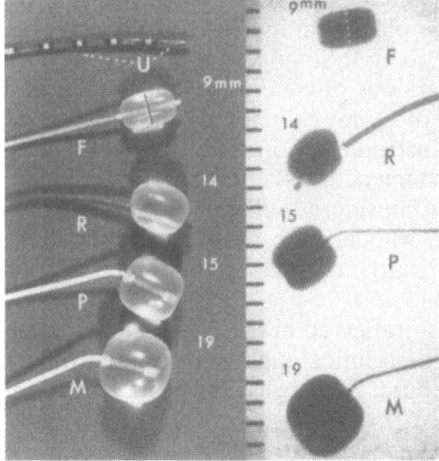

Fig. 7. Distended septostomy balloon catheters (recommended volumes) used for atrial septostomy. U, ureteral catheter similar to type used in Forssmann's selfcatheterization; F, Fogarty 4F embolectomy catheter (not an atrial septostomy catheter); R, Rashkind 5F atrial septostomy catheter; P, Fogarty (Paul) 5F dilation catheter for atrial septostomy; M, Miller (Fogarty) 6F balloon atrioseptostomy catheter (see Table 1.)

through multiple turns of the wire-winding, thus assuring maximum opportunity for balloon deflation; and 4) controlled proximal balloon windings such that the balloon, rather than rupture and fragment under excessive pull-force, will deflate by pulling out from under the proximal windings and evert over the distal tip.

This collaborative program brought forth the Fogarty (Paul) dilation catheter (Fig. 7, P) for atrial septostomy (1968) and, subsequently (1982), the larger balloon-volume Miller (Fogarty) balloon atrioseptostomy catheter (Fig. 7, M).

The mechanism of creating an atrial septostomy

In the newborn with transposition and intact ventricular septum, the septum primum flap forming the floor of the fossa ovalis is usually a quite thin, almost translucent membrane (Fig. 5, C_1). Premature closure of the foramen ovale which prevents a conventional septostomy has very rarely been noted in transposition newborns with intact ventricular septum, but is occassionally present in infants with large ventricular septal defects. At times, the septum primum flap, particularly in the older neonate with large ventricular septal defect, is a thicker, muscularized membrane (Fig. 5, C_2) that is not likely to tear with the pull-force of balloon septostomy. Such situations can be managed with the blade septostomy technique described by Park et al. [11].

Rashkind emphasized the need for a forceful and rapid tug and the use of an adequately sized balloon for the initial pull-through in an effort to not dilate the existing patent foramen ovale passage, but rather to create a tear in the septum primum flap.

For years, some have depicted the actual membrane rupture to occur as the balloon traverses the foramen ovale at the mid- or low-atrial level (Fig. 8). In our view, however, the rupture most often occurs after the contrast medium-filled balloon pulls the septum down onto the mouth of the inferior vena cava as illustrated in the high-speed recording from our laboratory (Fig. 9).

66

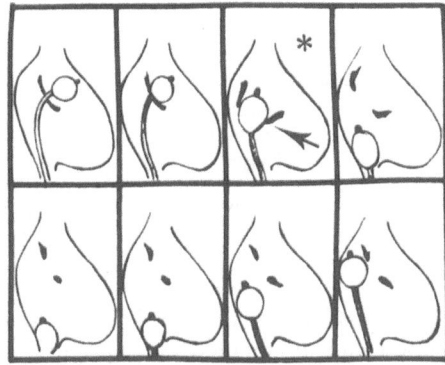

Fig. 8. Schematic drawing suggesting site and mechanism of septum primum valve tissue rupture (note frame with * and arrow) during balloon septostomy (reproduced from Rashkind [14]).

Possible causes for an unsuccessful clinical outcome of septostomy may be procedural, anatomical or physiological in nature. The former includes: inadequate balloon size, pull-force or pull-speed; thick septum primum membrane; premature closure or unusually small fossa ovalis (rare). Physiological causes of failure are related to suboptimal pulmonary blood flow and the resulting reduced pulmonary venous return and suboptimal interatrial mixing. In the absence of obvious *structural* left-ventricular outflow tract obstruction (LVOTO) this situation can be related to the infrequent occurrence of early, occult *dynamic* LVOTO [1] or to per-

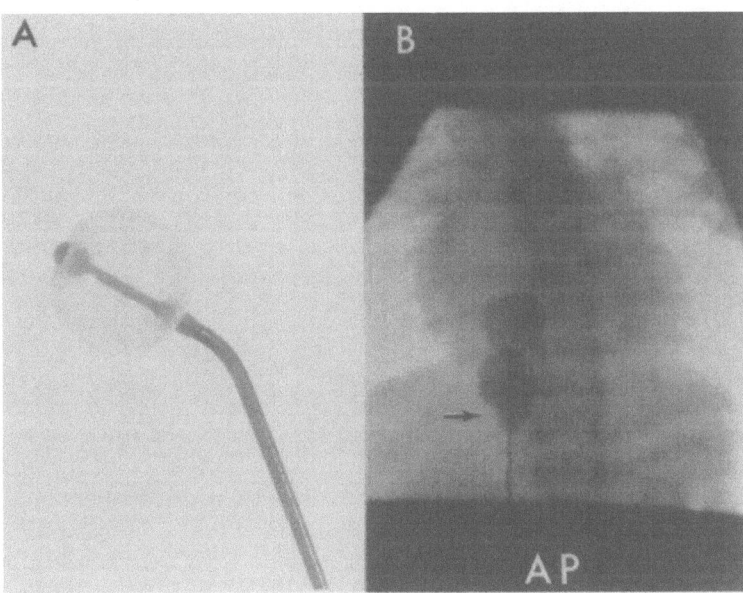

Fig. 9. Balloon atrial septostomy. A) 5F Fogarty dilation catheter distended to 15-mm diameter. B) High-speed (double-frame) cineangiogram of septostomy in neonate with transposition. Arrow indicates marked displacement of fossa ovalis segment with sudden, forceful pull-force. Note also the displacement of entire heart silhouette to right.

Table 2. Balloon atrial septostomy/atrial septal defect size

Patients (n)	Defect Size diameter	Defect size classification
23	<10 mm	small
27	10–15 mm	medium
40	>15 mm	Large

Assessment of atrial septal defect size after balloon atrial septostomy, made by balloon pull-through sizing at catheterization or measurement at surgery or autopsy.

sistent increased fetal pulmonary vascular vasoconstriction. Obviously, the impact of prostaglandin E_1 treatment and its associated transductal increase in pulmonary blood flow has favorably impacted this factor.

Atrial septal defect size after septostomy/criteria for satisfactory septostomy

We have reviewed reports attempting to relate the clinical and hemodynamic responses after septostomy to the size of the septostomy defect using observations from catherization (balloon-sizing), surgery, 2-D echocardiography, and autopsy. These findings suggest that a defect diameter of at least 12 mm, or more, is adequate when there are no pulmonary blood flow inhibitory factors present (Table 2). Indeed, the floor of the fossa ovalis in the newborn autopsy specimen rarely exceeds 12 to 15 mm in diameter (Fig. 10).

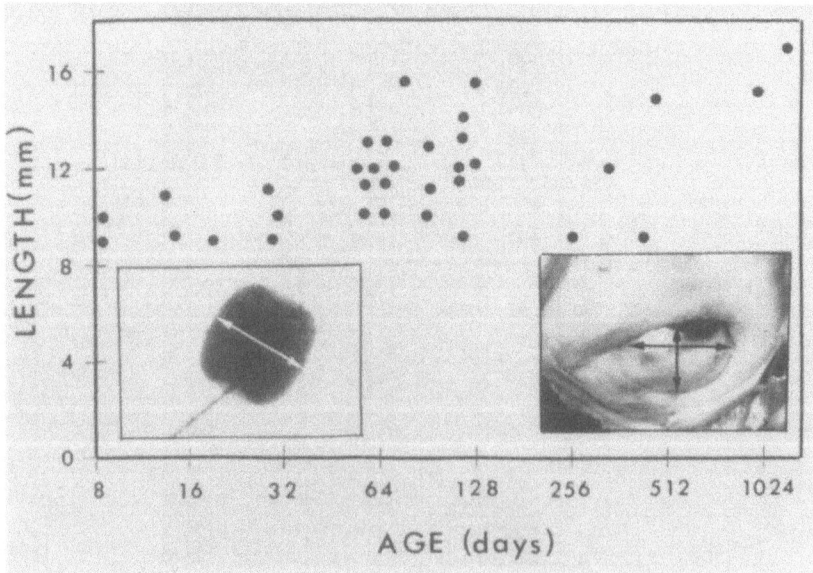

Fig. 10. Autopsy measurements of fossa ovalis in 34 patients with complete transposition. Age in days plotted on logarithmic (base 2) scale. Length (maximum) in millimeters, mm, without compensation for fixation shrinkage. (Reproduced with permission from Fisher EA, Paul MH (1970) Transposition of the great arteries: Recognition and management. Cardiovasc Clin 2:211–230.)

Table 3. Balloon atrial septostomy/TGA (IVS) systemic arterial oxygen saturation response*

Patients (n)	Oxygen saturation Pre-septostomy	Post-septostomy	Late follow-up
20	41%	64%	–
75	43 ± 12%	62 ± 12%	58 ± 9%
30	31 ± 11%	57 ± 12%	55 ± 10%

* Modified from Paul [10]
Systemic arterial oxygen (%) saturation response to septostomy in infants with transposition and intact ventricular septum (TGA-IVS).

In general, criteria for a satisfactory response to balloon atrial septostomy for transposition with intact ventricular septum included rapid clinical stabilization, increases in arterial saturation of about 20% (Table 3), and reduction in the inter-atrial mean pressure difference to less than 2 mmHg. With a large ventricular septal defect there may be little increase in arterial oxygen saturation, but left atrial pressure should decrease significantly.

Procedural complications have been infrequent but widely reported, and included rupture of the distended balloon with embolization of air bubbles or latex fragments, perforation of pulmonary vein or atrial chamber, atrioventricular valve damage, inferior vena caval tear, and balloon deflation failure.

Balloon atrial septostomy in the current era of arterial repair

In the current era of widespread and dramatic success with arterial repair for the neonate with transposition of the great arteries, the role of *routine atrial septostomy* is being actively reassessed. Indeed, sales statistics from catheter manufactures indicate a 50% decline in orders for septostomy catheters between 1987 and 1991.

For the neonate, immediate palliative support is usually provided by prostaglandin E_1 infusion and the diagnostic accuracy of 2-D and Doppler echocardiography is excellent. The status of the foramen ovale, ductus arteriosus, and proximal coronary arteries can be reliably assessed in the newborn patient [8]. A hemodynamically restrictive foramen ovale present in the minority of these infants (about 25%), can be readily identified with echo grading of the: a) interatrial septal bowing and bulging (Fig. 11); b) foramen ovale diameter; and c) transatrial Doppler flow velocity profiles. In these selected infants, who also fail to respond to prostaglandin E_1 therapy with a satisfactory increase in systemic arterial oxygenation (Table 4), balloon atrial septostomy may be necessary as an immediate support maneuver prior to arterial repair [2].

Conclusion

William J. Rashkind was a physician and scientist with immense spirit, enthusiasm, and talent-qualities manifest both in his work and his living. Quite simply, his involvement with the cardiac catheter *permanently altered the course of cardiology and opened the era of therapeutic interventional catheterization.*

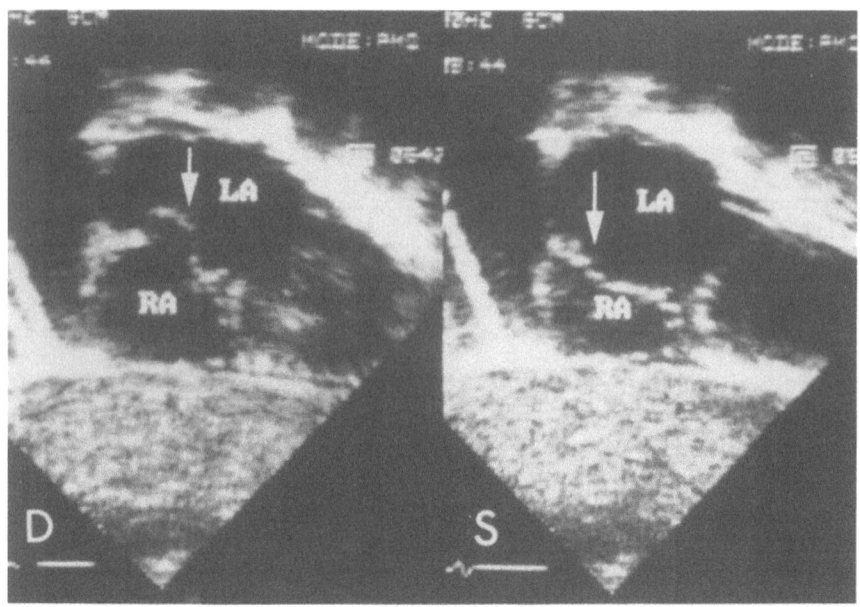

Fig. 11. Two-dimensional echocardiogram, subcostal view, in neonate with transposition and intact ventricular septum, demonstrating bowing and bulging of atrial septum (arrow), indicating restrictive foramen ovale with no significant interatrial mixing. D, diastole; LA, left and RA, right atrium; S, systole. (Reproduced by permission from [8].)

Table 4. TGA (IVS) / PGE$_1$ / Arterial repair*

BAS performed patients	(n)	Restrictive PFO (n)	Arterial PO$_2$ with PGE$_1$ torr	Arterial repair age (hours)	Survive arterial repair
No-BAS	12	0	43	36 h	12
Yes-Bas	3	3	preBAS 29 ▽ postBAS 43	148 h	2

* Modified from Baylen et al. [2]
Role of balloon atrial septostomy (BAS) in the current era for neonates with TGA-IVS. Three of 15 infants (Yes-BAS) had septostomy after 2-D echo-Doppler assessment indicated a restrictive foramen ovale. Note the mean arterial pO$_2$ achieved (43 torr) was the same as that present in the 12 No-BAS infants.

Acknowledgement

We are pleased to acknowledge the contributions of Dr. Henry R. Wagner, in particular, for providing the long-"lost" catheterization record (Fig. 6) of the first infant to have had a successful Rashkind balloon atrial septostomy; Dr. John A. Waldhausen for the recent late follow-up (after 26 years) information on this patient; Drs. William W. Miller and Sidney Friedman for observations about the initial experimental catheter constructions and clinical trials; Dennis C. Wood, Jr. research assistant and catheterization laboratory technician for observations (1971−1986); and catheter design engineers, Harvey Collins (USCI-Bard) and Clem Lieber (Edwards-Baxter Healthcare) for comments.

References

1. Aziz KU, Paul MH, Idriss FS, Wilson AJ, Muster AJ (1979) Clinical manifestations of dynamic left ventricular outflow tract stenosis with D-transposition of the great arteries with intact ventricular septum. Am J Cardiol 44:290−297
2. Baylen BG, Grzeszczak M, Gleason MM, Cyran SE, Weber HS, Meyers JL, Waldhausen JA (1990) Rashkind balloon atrial septostomy for cyanotic transposition of the great arteries. Is it always necessary? Ped Research 18:296 (abstr)
3. Blalock A, Hanlon CR (1950) The surgical treatment of complete transposition of the aorta and the pulmonary artery. Surg Gynecol Obstet 90:1−15
4. Cournand A, Baldwin JS, Himmelstein A (1949) Catheterization in congenital heart disease. The Commonwealth Fund, New York
5. Dotter CT, Judkins MP (1964) Transluminal treatment of arteriosclerotic obstruction. Circulation 30:654−670
6. Fogarty JT, Cranley JJ (1964) Catheter technique for arterial embolectomy. Ann Surg 161:325−330
7. Forssmann W (1929) Die Sondierung des rechten Herzens. Klin Wochenschr 8:2085−2087
8. Gotteiner NL, Duffy CE, Benson DW Jr, Sanders SP (1991) Preoperative echocardiographic assessment of D-transposition of the great arteries. In: Mavroudis C, Backer CL (eds) The Arterial Switch Operation, vol 5, number 1. Philadelphia, Hanley & Belfus, Inc., pp 83−98
9. Gruentzig AR (1978) Transluminal dilatation of coronary artery stenosis (Letter to the Editor). Lancet I:263
10. Paul MH (1989) Transposition of the Great Arteries. In: Heart Disease in Infants, Children, and Adolescents. 4th ed. Adams FH, Emmanoulides G, Riemenschneider TA (Eds) Williams & Wilkins, Baltimore p 371−423
11. Park SC, Neches WH, Zuberbuhler JR, Lenox CC, Matthews RA, Fricker FJ, Zoltun RA (1978) Clinical use of blade atrial septostomy. Circulation 58:600−606
12. Rashkind WJ (1954) Contributions of physiologic research to clinical cardiology. Med Clin North Am 38:565
13. Rashkind WJ (1963) Creation of an atrial defect without thoracotomy. Circulation 28:787 (abstr)
14. Rashkind WJ (1983) Transcatheter treatment of congenital heart disease. Circulation 67:711−716
15. Rashkind WJ, Miller WW (1966) Creation of an atrial septal defect without thoracotomy: A palliative approach to complete transposition of the great arteries. JAMA 196:991−992

Author's address:
Milton H. Paul, M.D.
The Willis J. Potts Children's Heart Center
The Children's Memorial Hospital
2300 Children's Plaza
Chicago, IL 60614, USA

Role of prostaglandin infusion prior to surgery in complete transposition of the great arteries

J. Kachaner
Hopital Necker-Enfants Malades, Paris, France

Introduction

The simple forms of transposition of the great arteries are not ductal dependent heart defects in a strict sense like pulmonary atresias. However, maintaining or restoring ductal patency may have a therapeutic effect in two ways in this congenital heart lesion.

Firstly, prostaglandins can be considered medical palliation, which may become necessary to improve mixing in cases with unfavorable hemodynamics. Although the mainstay of palliative intervention to improve mixing is the Rashkind balloon septostomy, prostaglandins may occasionally be indicated before or after the Rashkind maneuver.

Secondly, use of prostaglandins may be indicated in centers which have a protocol to repair complete transposition by anatomic correction with the arterial switch operation. Use of prostaglandins may alter volume loading of the left ventricle and thus aid in preserving (or restoring) its competence to serve as a systemic ventricle after the arterial switch operation.

These two important indications for use of prostaglandins in transposition will be discussed after review of some of the pertinent pathophysiological features of complete transposition of the great arteries.

Pathophysiology of complete transposition of the great arteries

After birth, survival of a neonate with transposition of the great arteries is only possible if there is some mixing of the "parallel circulations" [10]. This effectively occurs either via a patent ductus arteriosus or a patent foramen ovale, or if pulmonary venous and capillary pressures are elevated via bronchial arterial and venous communications. Independent of shunt site, the system is only hemodynamically balanced when the amount of blood passing from right to left is equal to the amount of blood passing in the opposite direction. Disturbance of this delicate balance may lead the patient to death.

In the common forms of simple transposition, the ductal shunt is bidirectional in the beginning, but develops into an aorto-pulmonary shunt when the pulmonary vascular resistance begins to fall. Increase of pulmonary blood flow will be balanced by a left to right shunt of the same magnitude either:

- through a foramen ovale, which may become dilated by increased pulmonary venous blood flow, causing distension of left atrium;

73

- through anastomoses between pulmonary veins and the azygos system caused by increased pulmonary venous pressure;
- through the patent duct itself, which may shunt left-to-right by altered post capillary resistance or pulmonary vasoconstriction.

In fact, all these mechanisms only contribute marginally to an increased shunt, which remains small, whereas the hypoxemia is a persistent clinical problem and development of pulmonary edema inevitably occurs. Thus, therapeutic intervention in the form of a septostomy is urgently indicated to increase atrial left-to-right shunting and balance the aorto-pulmonary shunt via the patent ductus. An effective Rashkind balloon septostomy thus creates a new balance with improved systemic oxygenation and decreased pulmonary pressures at the expense of volume-loading the right ventricle, whereas the left ventricle ejects a smaller blood volume against a lower pulmonary vascular resistance. The left-ventricular mass thus decreases and the left ventricle may finally lose its ability to function as a systemic ventricle [3].

Knowledge of these facts facilitates understanding of hemodynamic effects of prostaglandins in patients with transposition of the great arteries with regard to the two indications mentioned above. Besides having a potent effect on the arterial duct [5], prostaglandins have multiple side-effects which are listed in Table 1. The most important one is the occurrence of apneas in up to 30% of patients, which may necessitate artificial ventilation [8].

Table 1. Side-effects of intravenous PGE1

- Localized vasodilation (flush)
- Generalized vasodilation (collapse)
- Minor arrhythmias
- Fever (moderate)
- Seizures (?)
- Infections (?)
- Gastro-intestinal problems (?)
- Renal dysfunction (?)
- Clotting problems (?)

- APNEAS → BRADYCARDIA or CARDIAC ARREST

(?) = questionable direct relationship

Prostaglandins as palliative drugs in simple transposition of the great arteries in the neonate

Use of prostaglandins has been advocated since the late 1970s to improve mixing in patients with transposition of the great vessels after balloon septostomy either had not or only marginally improved mixing, or this improvement had only been transitory [2, 4, 5, 6, 7]. The use of prostaglandins *after* balloon septostomy has usually been effective, if the arterial duct had not been irreversibly closed and if pulmonary vascular resistance had been low enough to allow for a significant aorto-pulmonary shunt leading to an increase in atrial left-to-right shunt, as was mentioned above.

Usually, risk of development of pulmonary edema is low or absent if a good intra-atrial communication was previously achieved by Rashkind balloon septostomy. Use of prostaglandins after balloon septostomy has obviated the need for a second balloon septostomy or surgical septectomy in many cases [2, 7].

The use of prostaglandins *before* balloon septostomy is more complex and carries potential risks. If the foramen ovale is congenitally relatively large, then dilatation of the patent ductus is advantageous in that it increases pulmonary venous return, even though it may lead to a significant intraatrial pressure gradient [1]. In cases of very small and restrictive foramen ovale the excess pulmonary venous return may not egress the left atrium and may subsequently lead to severe pulmonary edema, which may become life-threatening.

This is the reason why we recommend to other hospitals making referrals to us not to start prostaglandins if the neonate is stable but cyanotic, and if the center does not have the ability to examine the intraatrial septum by echocardiography. In contrast, we recommend use of prostaglandins if the neonate is in an unstable hemodynamic condition with acidosis, but we stress the need of a speedy transfer to a specialized center where a Rashkind balloon septostomy can be performed.

Use of prostaglandins to prepare the left ventricle before anatomic correction of transposition in the neonate

Anatomic correction by arterial switch operation can be successfully achieved in the first 15 days of life, as long as the left ventricle still has the capability to function as a systemic ventricle [11]. In the fetus and during the first days of life both ventricles in complete transposition have a similar afterload to handle and have a similar myocardial mass. During the following weeks, however, the subaortic morphologically right ventricle has a much higher workload than the subpulmonary morphologically left ventricle, which loses its "systemic competence" (Fig. 1). Serial

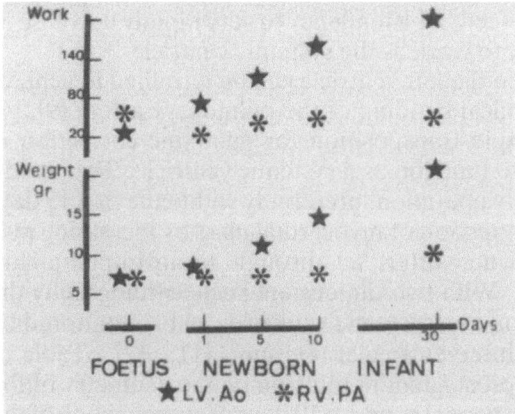

Fig. 1. Right- and left-ventricular weight and work before and after birth (experimental work in sheep fetuses and lambs, unpublished data). Stars: left ventricle (subaortic), Asterisks: right ventricle (subpulmonary)

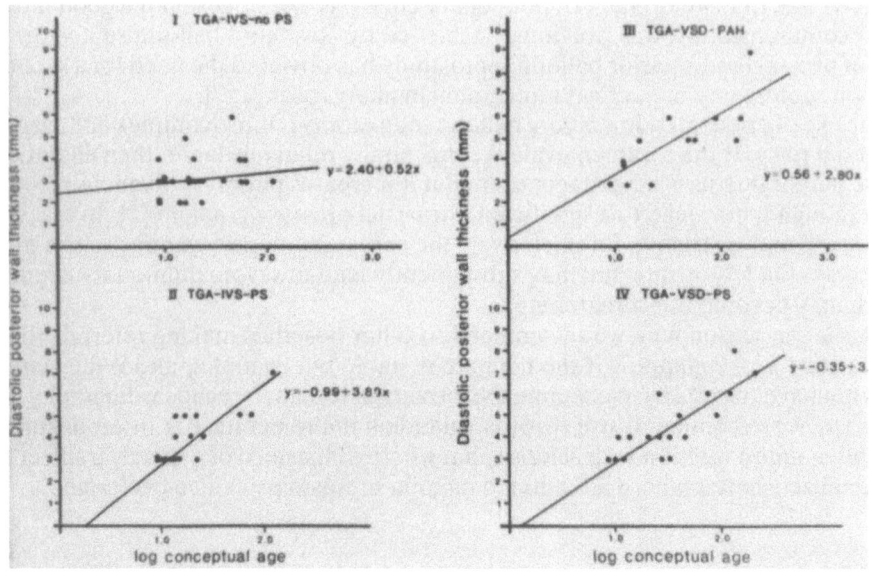

Fig. 2. Left-ventricular diastolic posterior wall thickness in patients with transposition of the great arteries (TGA) (from [2]). Group I: intact ventricular septum (IVS) and no pulmonary stenosis (PS), Group II: IVS and PS, Group III: ventricular septal defect (VSD) and pulmonary artery hypertension (PAH), Group IV: VSD and PS. The rate of increase of Group I is significantly lower than rates in the other three groups (p < 0.05)

echocardiographic studies in Houston [3] with different types of transposition of the great vessels have confirmed these assumptions. Figure 2 illustrates that the left ventricle in simple transposition with intact ventricular septum compared to forms of transposition of the great arteries associated with increased left-ventricular afterload, either by the presence of pulmonary stenosis with or without intact ventricular septum or increased pulmonary vascular resistance due to a significant shunt through a ventricular septal defect, has a tendency to very rapidly decrease its myocardial mass and lose the ability to work as the systemic ventricle.

Aside from those patients in whom the left ventricle can be retrained to achieve systemic workload by means of surgical banding of the pulmonary artery [9], we should consider those cases of simple transposition for anatomic correction in whom the left ventricle is still able to function as a systemic ventricle. Two conditions have to be fulfilled: first an early operation, preferably within the first 15 days of life; and second, prevention of regression of myocardial mass by increasing pulmonary blood flow and left-ventricular afterload through an aorto-pulmonary shunt via a patent ductus arteriosus. With two-dimensional echocardiography the ability of the left ventricle to function as a systemic ventricle can be monitored by assessing the geometry of the interventricular septum [11, 12]. Table 2 demonstrates the effect of age and prostaglandin infusion on the geometry of the interventricular septum. None of the neonates under 10 days of age and none of the infants with prostaglandin infusion had an unfavorable septal geometry, whereas this could be observed in infants older than 10 days and those not having received prostaglandins.

Table 2. Influence of age and PGE1 infusion on left-ventricular geometry in 54 neonates with simple transposition of great arteries

	No. of cases	Septal geometry assessed by 2D echo		
		Favorable	Intermediate	Unfavorable
2– 9 days	40	25	15	0
10–23 days	14	3	9	2
with PGE1	45	28	17	0
without PGE1	9	0	7	2

Table 3. Pre-operative management in 220 neonates with simple tgransposition of the great arteries (Paris, 1984–1991)

- Balloon atrioseptostomy: 190 (86%)
- PGE1 infusion: 200 (91%)
  - maintained: 176
  - discontinued: 24
- Artificial ventilation: 90 (41%)
  (more than 2 days)

Table 4. Current prostaglandin protocol in neonates with simple transposition of the great arteries (Paris, April 1991)

- Atrial septal defect should be checked as Non Restrictive (natural anatomy or after balloon atrioseptostomy)

  - Infuse prostaglandin E1 (Prostin VR°)
  - IV route, constant flow, 5% glucose
  - 0.1 to 0.025 mcg/kg/mn

  - Artificial ventilation if apneas
  - Withdraw if cardiac failure due to high left-right ductal flow

Taking into account these data, a management protocol for neonates with transposition of the great arteries and intact ventricular septum should consist of: 1) obligatory Rashkind balloon septostomy to protect the neonate from a possibly fatal pulmonary edema, 2) prostaglandin infusion to achieve or maintain ductal patency and thus increase pulmonary blood flow and left-ventricular work load and, 3) anatomic correction by arterial switch operation, preferably in the first week of life and before the end of the second week of life at the latest.

This management protocol has been altered with time and experience and can be modified to take into account the anatomical and physiological variations in individual neonates with transposition, as both balloon septostomy and prostaglandin infusion may carry some (albeit small) risks. Table 3 shows that a Rashkind balloon septostomy has not been performed in 14% of our neonates with simple transposition. Those neonates either had an adequate shunt at atrial level as assessed by clinical status and echocardiography, or they were operated very early. However, these neonates have to be closely monitored and one has to be prepared to perform balloon septostomy on an emergency basis at any time. Prostaglandin infusion can be withheld if the ductus is widely patent with a significant aorto-pulmonary shunt and if left-ventricular shape is and rests favorable up to the point of surgical intervention. In 12% of our cases, we stopped the prostaglandin infusion because the neonates developed signs of congestive heart failure (Table 4).

In conclusion, the objective of preoperative management of a neonate with simple transposition is to preserve the neonate's life in the best possible hemodynamic condition. The Rashkind balloon septostomy is very helpful to achieve this goal, but it may not be necessary in those neonates who have clinical and echocardiographic evidence of an adequate atrial shunt and can be surgically corrected within a few days. After the first few days, only neonates with evidence of adequate left ventricle should be proposed for an arterial switch. Prostaglandin infusion may be needed to increase left-ventricular workload, but it can probably be omitted and its serious side effects (apneas, risk of congestive heart failure) can be avoided if anatomic correction is performed within the first 15 days of life or if septal geometry suggests suitability of the left ventricle to support the systemic circulation.

References

1. Beitzke A, Suppan CH (1983) Use of prostaglandin E2 in management of transposition of great arteries before balloon atrial septostomy. Br Heart J 49:341–344
2. Benson LN, Olley PM, Patel RG, Coceani F, Rowe RD (1979) Role of prostaglandin E1 in the management of transposition of the great arteries. Am J Cardiol 44:591–696
3. Danford DA, Huhta JC, Gutgesell HP (1985) Left ventricular wall stress and thickness in complete transposition of the great arteries. Implications for surgical intervention. J Thorac Cardiovasc Surg 89:610–615
4. Driscoll DJ, Kugler JD, Nihill MR, McNamara DG (1979) The use of prostaglandin E1 in a critically ill infant with transposition of the great arteries. J Pediatr 95:259–261
5. Freed MD, Heymann MA, Lewis AB, Roehl SL, Kensey RC (1981) Prostaglandin E1 in infants with ductus arteriosus dependent congenital heart disease. Circulation 64:899–905
6. Henry CG, Goldring D, Hartmann AF, Weldon CS, Strauss AW (1981) Treatment of d-transposition of the great arteries: management of hypoxemia after balloon atrial septostomy. Am J Cardiol 47:299–306
7. Lang P, Freed MD, Bierman FZ, Norwood WI, Nadas AS (1979) Use of prostaglandin E1 in infants with d-transposition of the great arteries and intact ventricular septum. Am J Cardiol 44:76–81
8. Lewis AB, Freed MD, Heymann MA, Roehl SL, Kensey RC (1981) Side-effects of therapy with prostaglandin E1 in infants with critical congenital heart disease. Circulation 64:893–898
9. Sidi D, Heurtematte Y, Kachaner J, Fermont L, Batisse A, Villain E, Hazan E, Lecompte Y (1983) Problèmes posés par la préparation du ventricule gauche à la correction anatomique de la transposition des gros vaisseaux. Arch Mal Coeur 76:575–583
10. Sidi D, Heymann MA (1984) Physiopathologie de la transposition des gros vaisseaux. Ann Pédiatr 31:529–532
11. Sidi D, Planché C, Kachaner J, Bruniaux J, Villain E, Le Bibois J, Piéchaud JF, Lacour-Gayet F (1987) Anatomic correction of simple transposition of the great arteries in 50 neonates. Circulation 75:429–435
12. Van Doesburg NH, Bierman FZ, Williams RG (1983) Left ventricular geometry in infants with d-transposition of the great arteries and intact ventricular septum. Circulation 68:733–739

Author's address:
Dr. Jean Kachaner
Hopital Necker-Enfants Malades
149 Rue de Sevres
75743 Paris Cedex 15
France

78

The natural history of transposition after balloon septostomy and before surgical repair

M. Tynan, E. J. Baker, S. Qureshi, E. Rosenthal, A. Kakadeker
Guy's Hospital London, England

Introduction

Prior to the introduction of balloon atrial septostomy [12] the mortality of infants with transposition was high, even with state-of-the-art palliation [5]. Undoubtedly, Rashkind's innovation resulted in a revolutionary change in outlook for such infants. What is more, it came at a time when this improvement could be exploited to maximum effect due to the introduction and widespread success of the Mustard procedure for atrial redirection of venous return [10, 1]. Early in the experience of the use of balloon atrial septostomy the results seemed so self-evidently good [13] that little attention was paid to factors which might determine survival and thus might be influenced to improve outcome. Haemodynamic improvement was talked of in terms of percentage increase in arterial oxygen saturation and was not further analysed until some 6 years had passed. By this time, it had become evident that anatomical factors influenced the effect on arterial oxygenation and physiological influences were being sought. By the early 1970s we understood that the most dramatic increases in arterial saturation were seen in those with the poorest natural anatomical sites for intracirculatory mixing. In fact, the effect on the population of infants was to convert the two populations of 'poor mixers' and 'good mixers' into one population of better mixers [6]. Despite the improvements in haemodynamics and early survival there was a continuous attrition, and survival at 30 months was of the order of 50% [14].

Factors influencing survival

In the hands of experienced operators the procedure was, and still is, extremely safe. In the series of 80 patients that formed the body of my doctoral thesis there was only death directly related to the procedure and this was unexplained at autopsy. There were no incidental intracardiac injuries in this group. Deaths in the early years of balloon atrial septostomy centred on thromboembolic complications suffered whilst awaiting definitive surgery. As the age for the Mustard procedure was progressively lowered further improvements in overall survival were obtained. But even with surgery at 6 months of age not all infants had survived. Analysis of the influences on survival identified some beneficial factors, such as initial high interatrial pressure gradient or high arterial oxygen saturation. These factors, although improving the chances of survival, reflected the state of the infant before septostomy and, thus before admission to the paediatric cardiology service; there was, therefore, little that could be done to alter them [7]. Leanage and his colleagues in 1981 [9] analysed 144 patients to investigate risk factors for death

Table 1. Transposition of the great arteries. Age at presentation to the paediatric cardiology service in two eras, 1966–1970 and 1980–1988

Age	1966–1970		1980–1988	
Prenatal	0		1	1.2%
1st day of life	4	5%	40	54%
2–8 days	20	25%	23	31.4%
8–28 days	27	34%	9	12.1%
1–3 months	19	24%	1	1.2%
over 3 months	10	12%	0	
Total	80		74	

between septostomy and definitive surgery, ideally performed at around 6 months of age. They were interested in defining the conditions in the postseptostomy phase which might be influenced to improve survival. Many of their conclusions make sense whilst some do not. Thromboembolic complications were confirmed as an important cause of death whilst awaiting surgery. This was in line with a previous report from the same unit where 10 of 80 patients had suffered such events [14]. In fact, these patients were included in Leanage's analysis, so this agreement is not surprising. Other factors included the effect of septostomy on the arterial oxygen saturation where a small rise was less beneficial than a large one or better than no rise at all. This can probably be explained on the basis that no rise meant that there were anatomical sites for mixing before septostomy and that the saturation could not be expected to increase, whilst a large rise indicated little anatomical possibility for mixing before the procedure [6].

More importantly, the long-term level of arterial oxygenation was optimal at a PO_2 of 25 to 45 mmHg. A higher value being associated with, for example, a ventricular septal defect which carried a cost in terms of high pulmonary blood flow and, often, pulmonary hypertension, itself an independent risk factor. In addition to the presence of a large ventricular septal defect other anatomical lesions predisposing to death included coarctation of the aorta and aortic stenosis. There is little to argue about in the incrimination of these additional anomalies. However, they found that the absence of left-ventricular outflow obstruction predisposed to death. This is a bit difficult to explain, in the absence of an associated ventricular septal defect. Furthermore, they identified a persistent arterial duct, even a small one, as a disadvantageous factor. This was the one anatomical lesion that it was possible to influence since, in general, it was not the policy to close small ducts surgically and they implicitly recommend closure. The beneficial effects of prostaglandin therapy seem to be in contrast to this conclusion. Of the other factors, the most important is the adverse effect of relative anaemia. This, at least, we can prevent by careful haematological monitoring. Finally, the outcome was influenced by the era of and the age at septostomy. Survival to 6 months improved from 55% before December 1972 to 74% in the period 1973 through 1975, whilst from 1976 onwards there was a further improvement to 86%. Moreover, there was an increased mortality when septostomy was performed between 1 week and 1 month of age. That is to say that delay in septostomy after 1 week in those with poor mixing was a bad thing. The independence of these observations may not be complete. Delay in septostomy was not due to infants waiting in the cardiology service, but due to delay in diagnosis or to delay in admission to the specialized centre. By 1978, most diagnoses of congenital heart disease were established by 1 week to 1 month of age [8]. That this was previously the case is illustrated in Table 1, which contrasts the ages at which septostomy was performed at The Hospital for Sick Children, Great Ormond Street prior to 1971, with similar data from Guy's Hospital since 1977. We see that the majority were treated after 1 week of age in the earlier series, whereas the converse is true in the latter group. Thus, era of and age at septostomy are related. This improvement in the speed of referral may reflect changes in awareness of neonatologists, but also is due to the wider availability of specialised facilities.

Balloon atrial septostomy today

The arterial-switch operation is now the procedure of choice in the newborn period [11] and, thus, the indications for balloon septostomy are now different; however, this aspect is outside the scope of this article. Today, the technique has been modified. The demonstration that the procedure could be performed under cross-sectional echocardiographic control [2] has allowed the transfer of the procedure from the catheter laboratory to the intensive care unit [3]. The use of echocardiography makes the identification of the balloon in the left atrium more secure at the start of the pullback and makes easier confirmation that the atrial septum has been crossed, and torn, at the completion of the pullback. Today, even those rare accidents during septostomy should be eliminated. We have analysed the data from 60 consecutive patients (pts) with transposition (58 pts) or double-outlet right ventricle with subpulmonary ventricular septal defect (2 pts) treated in the intensive care unit from our initiation of this approach up to April 1981. In all, five patients died between the septostomy and definitive surgery, a survival rate of 92%. Three deaths which occurred in the initial admission were due to necrotizing enterocolitis in two, and in one there was persistent severe hypoxaemia despite an anatomically adequate interatrial defect. Of equal importance was the fact that only one patient suffered a thromboembolic episode; he survived the stroke and is alive, having made a good neurological recovery.

These results demonstrate the safety of 'bedside' balloon septostomy. In addition, it can be done without waiting for a space in the catheter room schedule or for calling in the on-call catheter staff, thus minimising delays and reducing costs, all factors which have led to its popularity [4]. However, the improvement in survival cannot be attributed to this change alone. Ten of our patients needed prostaglandin E^2 treatment for longer than 2 weeks and three were ventilated for prostaglandin-induced apnoea. Nonetheless, when required, balloon atrial septostomy can now be performed with a speed and safety unthought of by Rashkind 25 years ago.

References

1. Aberdeen E, Waterston DJ, Carr I, Graham G, Bonham-Carter RE, Subramanian S (1965) Successful 'correction' of transposed great arteries by Mustard's operation. Lancet II:1233–1235
2. Allan LD, Leanage R, Wainright R, Joseph MC, Tynan M (1982) Balloon atrial septostomy under two-dimensional echocardiographic control. Br Heart J 47:41–43

3. Baker EJ, Allan LD, Tynan MJ, Jones ODH, Joseph MC, Deverall PB (1984) Balloon atrial septostomy in the neonatal intensive are unit. Br Heart J 51:377–378
4. Beitzke A, Stein JL, Suppan C (1991) Balloon atrial septostomy under two dimensional echocardiographic control. Int J Cardiol 30:33–42
5. Deverall PB, Tynan M, Carr I, Panagopoulis P, Aberdeen E, Bonham-Carter RE, Waterston DJ (1969) Palliative surgery in children with transposition of the great arteries. J Thorac Cardiovasc Surg 58:721–729
6. Tynan M (1972) Haemodynamic effects of balloon atrial septostomy in infants with transposition of the great arteries. Br Heart J 34:791–794
7. Hawker RE, Krovetz LJ, Rowe RD (1974) An analysis of prognostic features in the outcome of balloon atrial septostomy for transposition of the great arteries. Johns Hopkins Med J 134:95–106
8. Hoffman JIE, Christianson R (1978) Congenital heart disease in a cohort of 19,502 births with long-term follow-up. Am J Cardiol 42:641–647
9. Leanage R, Agnetti A, Graham G, Taylor J, Macartney FJ (1981) Factors influencing survival after balloon atrial septostomy for complete transposition of great arteries. Br Heart J 45:559–572
10. Mustard WJ, Keith JD, Trussler GA, Fowler R, Kidd L (1964) The surgical management of transposition of the great vessels. J Thorac Cardiovasc Surg 48:953–958
11. Quaegebeur J, Rohmer J, Ottencamp J et al. (1986) The arterial switch operation – an eight year experience. J Thorac Cardiovasc Surg 92:361–384
12. Rashkind WJ, Miller WW (1966) Creation of atrial septal defect without thoracotomy. JAMA 196:991–992
13. Rashkind WJ, Miller WW (1968) Transposition of the great arteries. Results of palliation by balloon atrioseptostomy in thirty-one infants. Circulation 38:453–455
14. Tynan M (1977) Survival of infants with transposition of the great arteries after balloon atrial septostomy. Lancet I:622–623

Author's address:
Prof. Dr. M. Tynan
Department of Paediatric Cardiology
Guy's Hospital
London SE1 9RT
UK.

The natural history of the patient with transposition of the great arteries before atrial septostomy

R. M. Freedom
The University of Toronto Faculty of Medicine, The Hospital for Sick Children, Toronto, Canada

Dr. Bühlmeyer, distinguished colleagues, ladies and gentlemen:
I am singularly honored and delighted to be here in Munich, and to participate in this symposium dedicated to the life and contributions of the late William J. Rashkind. How fitting this festival of learning is conducted in Munich, because Bill Rashkind was a great traveller, one who appreciated art and history, philosophy, and friends. It is particularly appropriate that this symposium is held in 1991, 25 years after the introduction of the balloon atrial septostomy. How this technique forever changed the fortunes, indeed, the tapestry of the patient with complete transposition of the great arteries.

For those engaged in the care of the child with congenital heart disease, one of the greatest dramas of the past three decades is the changing fortune of the patient with complete transposition of the great arteries. The tapestry of this disorder is particularly rich, with an elegant background of cardiac anatomy, physiology, cardiac imaging with angiography of the 1950s and the early 1960s, and the emphasis on an appropriate way of designating hearts where the ventriculoarterial connection was so clearly disordered. But that rich and colored foreground was overshadowed by the reality of the disorder: survival and life-expectancy for the patient with complete transposition of the great arteries before the modern era of therapy was limited to those patients with naturally-occurring sites for intra- or extracardiac mixing. Data provided by Liebman et al. [3] showed that more than 80% of patients with transposition of the great arteries were dead by 1 year of age, and even for those few patients surviving to 1 year of age, survival to only about 3.9 years could be anticipated. These data are not surprising when one remembers that about 75% of patients have an intact ventricular septum (or nearly so); 15–20% a large ventricular septal defect; about 5%, ventricular septal and important left-ventricular outflow tract obstruction; and 1–2%, transposition of the great arteries, an intact ventricular septum and important left-ventricular outflow tract obstruction. What did these patients die from? Hypoxemia, congestive heart failure, infection, and surgery, the last usually performed to augment mixing between the systemic venous and pulmonary venous circulations.

Some patients with transposition would survive past the first few months of life.

Table 1. Types of transposition surviving the neonatal period

- TGA and large ASD
- TGA and large VSD
- TGA and large PDA
- TGA, VSD, and mild moderate, LVOTO

The list in Table 1 includes the patient with naturally-occurring large atrial septal defect, large ventricular septal defect: large patent arterial duct; and some patients with transposition, ventricular septal defect, and mild-to-modest left ventricular outflow tract obstruction. For those babies surviving the neonatal period with large VSD or patent arterial duct, congestive heart failure and early-onset pulmonary vascular obstructive disease were particularly common life (or death) events.

Interwoven with the tapestry of the disease are a number of interventions designed to improve the quality of life of these patients. The benchmark contributions to the treatment of the patient with complete transposition of the great arteries include:

1) The Senning operation, 1959 [2].
2) The Mustard operation, 1963 [3].
3) Balloon atrial septostomy, Rashkind and Miller, 1964 [4].
4) The arterial switch with coronary transfer of Jatene, 1974 [5].

It is of interest that the first two of these signal contributions were both atrial switch or inflow operations [5, 6], achieving a physiologic repair, rather than an anatomic one, and while the natural history of the patient with complete transposition of the great arteries would forever be altered by these venous switch operations, they still carried in the early-mid 1960s significant mortality, particularly the Senning operation, which rapidly fell into disfavor until its resurgence in the mid 1970s. Both Senning and Mustard probably assimilated and indeed benefited from the experience of Albert, Baffes, Blalock, Hanlon, and others who tried partial venous switches and atrial septal defect creation in the patient with transposition.

Table 2. Surgical procedures important in the history of transposition:

- Blalock-Hanlon
- Albert procedure
- Baffes procedure
- Senning procedure
- Mustard procedure
- Jatene arterial switch

But in the 1960s the venous repairs listed in Table 2 were not performed in the neonate or the young baby and, thus, there was continuing loss of life until the patients were considered old and large enough for an atrial switch operation (often 1 year of age or older). This all changed with the introduction of balloon atrial septostomy, one of the many important contributions of William J. Rashkind. The ability to non-surgically create an atrial septal defect is one of those special contributions of genius: obvious and simple to apply. But that is the stuff of Bill Rashkind. Other speakers in this symposium will address the fate of the patient after the Rashkind balloon atrial septostomy. Suffice it to say, this technique has now been extended to a wide range of congenitally malformed hearts where an obligatory shunt at atrial level (right-to-left or left-to-right) is necessary. The application of this technique forever changed the lifetable and survival statistics for the

84

patient with complete transposition of the great arteries. For the neonate with complete transposition of the great arteries and normal coronary arteries, we anticipate a Kaplan-Meier survival curve of more than 90% at 10 years of life.

But one should remember that even after the balloon septostomy technique was introduced and became integrated as standard therapy for the neonate with complete transposition of the great arteries, a few babies still died before balloon septostomy could be applied. Data from Trusler and the Hospital for Sick Children in Toronto [10] and Louhimo from Helsinki provide an incidence of 3–7% dying before balloon atrial septostomy could be accomplished.

Today, before balloon atrial septostomy is applied, the usual attention to normothermia, prevention of hypoglycemia, treatment of metabolic acidosis, ventilation with paralysis to reduce oxygen demands, and the administration of an E-type prostaglandin [1] all may serve to improve the hypoxemic baby prior to the performance of balloon atrial septostomy (Table 3).

Table 3. Medical adjuncts in the treatment of the newborn with TGA

- Maintenance of normothermia
- Prevention of hypoglycemia
- Treatment of acidemia
- Ventilation/paralysis to reduce oxygen requirements
- Administration of E-type prostaglandin

As with the administration of any medication, an E-type prostaglandin, both by promoting pulmonary vasodilatation and ductal patency, may result in pulmonary edema in those instances where the interatrial septum is nearly intact.

In closing, while we are celebrating the man (William J. Rashkind) and his contribution (Balloon atrial septostomy) [6–8], it is ironic that with the introduction of the arterial switch with coronary transfer as the procedure of choice for the neonate with transposition of the great arteries, balloon atrial septostomy is no longer performed for some patients with complete transposition of the great arteries. Knowing Bill Rashkind, he would smile at this irony.

References

1. Beitzke A, Suppan CH (1983) Use of prostaglandin E2 in management of transposition of great arteries before balloon atrial septostomy. Br Heart J 49:341–344
2. Jatene AD, Fontes VF, Paulista PP, Souza LCB, Neger F, Galantier M, Sousa JEMR (1976) Anatomic correction of transposition of the great vessels. J Thorac Cardiovasc Surg 72:364–370
3. Liebman J, Cullum L, Belloc NB (1969) Natural history of transposition of the great arteries. Anatomy and birth and death characteristics. Circulation XL:237–262
4. Louhimo I (1985) Complete transposition in Finland. Int J Cardiol 8:261–265
5. Mustard WT (1964) Successful two-stage correction of transposition of the great vessels. Surgery 55:469–472
6. Rashkind WJ, Miller WW (1966) Creation of an atrial septal defect without thoracotomy. A palliative approach to complete transposition of the great arteries. JAMA 196:991–992
7. Rashkind WJ (1974) Balloon atrioseptostomy. Adv Cardiol 11:2–10

8. Rashkind WJ (1983) Balloon atrioseptostomy revisited: the first fifteen years. Int J Cardiol 4:369–372
9. Senning A (1959) Surgical correction of transposition of the great vessels. Surgery 45:966–980
10. Trusler GA, Gonzales JC, Craig BG, Williams WG, Freedom RM, Rowe RD (1986) Isolated transposition of the great arteries: the present unnatural history. In: Doyle EF, Engle MA, Gersony WM, Rashkind WJ, Talner NS (eds) Paediatric Cardiology. Springer, New York, pp 1315–1319

Author's address:
Robert M. Freedom, M.D.
The University of Toronto
Faculty of Medicine
Division of Cardiology
The Hospital for Sick Children
Toronto, Canada

The pulmonary circulation in transposition of the great arteries

S. G. Haworth
Hospital for Sick Children, London

In the days before a Rashkind septostomy the average life-expectancy was 1.3 months in babies with transposition of the great arteries (TGA) and an intact ventricular septum (IVS), and 3.4 months in those with a TGA and ventricular septal defect (VSD) [14]. Those with a VSD survived longer because mixing of the pulmonary and systemic circulations persisted after closure of the foramen ovale and ductus arteriosus. A high effective pulmonary blood flow ensures a greater systemic arterial oxygen saturation. The presence of a large VSD however, leads to the rapid development of severe pulmonary vascular disease [6, 17]. In the presence of an intact ventricular septum a patent ductus arteriosus also leads to the early development of pulmonary vascular disease and should be closed surgically at 3 months of age if it has not already closed spontaneously. In transposition as a whole, patient outcome correlates with the pulmonary arterial pressure [13]. The outlook for patients with an IVS was transformed by the introduction of the Senning operation in 1959 and the Mustard repair in 1964, but not until the revival of the arterial switch procedure in 1976 did the long-term outlook improve for those with a VSD [16, 18, 20, 21, 22]. This procedure enables an early repair to be carried out with an acceptable risk, before severe pulmonary vascular disease has developed.

In the presence of an intact ventricular septum the pulmonary circulation usually adapts normally to extrauterine life. The endothelial and smooth muscle cells of the peripheral thickwalled pulmonary arteries become thin and spread within the vessel wall to achieve a reduction in wall thickness and an increase in lumen diameter without there being a reduction in the amount of pulmonary vascular smooth muscle (Fig. 1). The bronchial circulation is enlarged, and angiography suggests that the bronchial flow is high from birth (Fig. 2). This would not be surprising since communications between the pulmonary and bronchial circulations are normally larger in the fetus and newborn than later. The bronchial circulation makes a large but unknown contribution to total pulmonary blood flow. An enlarged bronchial circulation can sometimes persist after a successful intracardiac repair. Today nearly all patients with TGA and IVS undergo intracardiac repair with a relatively normal pulmonary vasculature. In the days before an intracardiac repair could be carried out in early infancy children developed severe polycythemia and thromboembolic changes were seen in the lungs.

In the presence of a large VSD the pulmonary vasculature does not remodel normally after birth and this failure to remodel marks the onset of pulmonary vascular obstructive disease [7]. In the presence of a high pulmonary arterial pressure the muscular pulmonary arteries are abnormally thick-walled and muscle extends into smaller, more peripheral arteries than normal. The media hypertrophies by an increase in size and number of smooth muscle cells and by deposition of excessive amounts of connective tissue [7]. The elastic lamellae become abnormally thick,

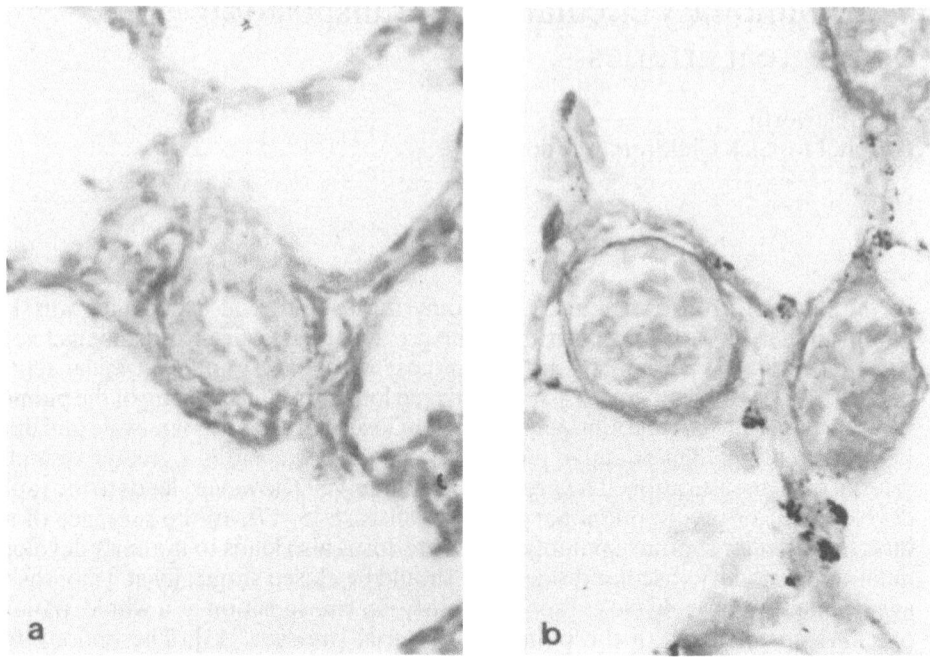

Fig. 1. Photomicrographs showing peripheral pulmonary arteries which are a) thick-walled at birth and, in the same baby, b) thin-walled at 2.5 months of age.

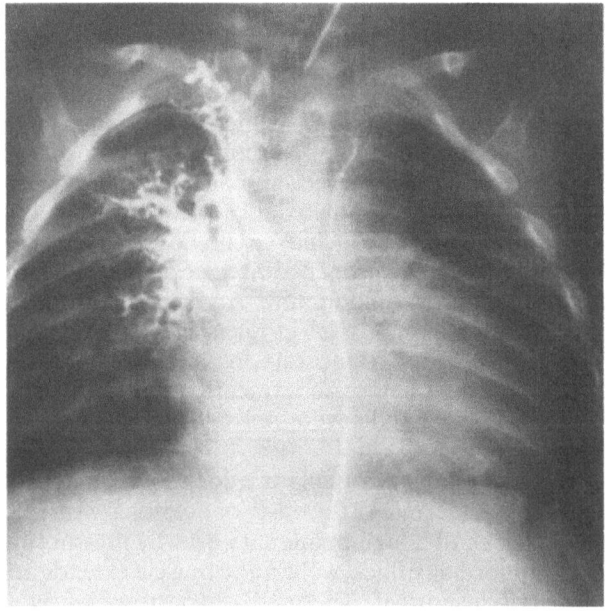

Fig. 2. Transposition of the great arteries with intact ventricular septum: angiogram showing enlarged bronchial arterial circulation following an otherwise successful Senning operation.

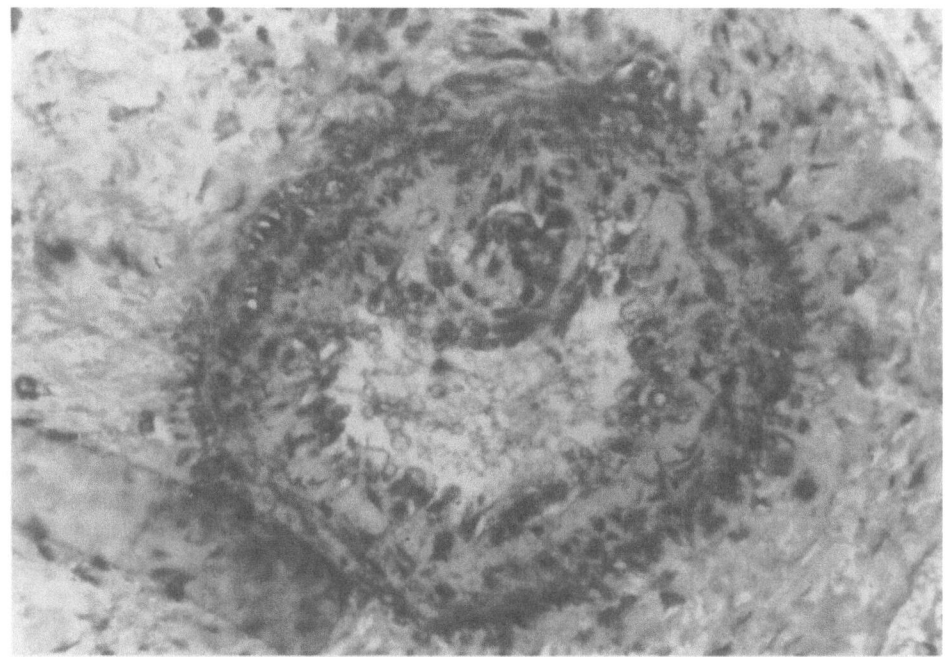

a

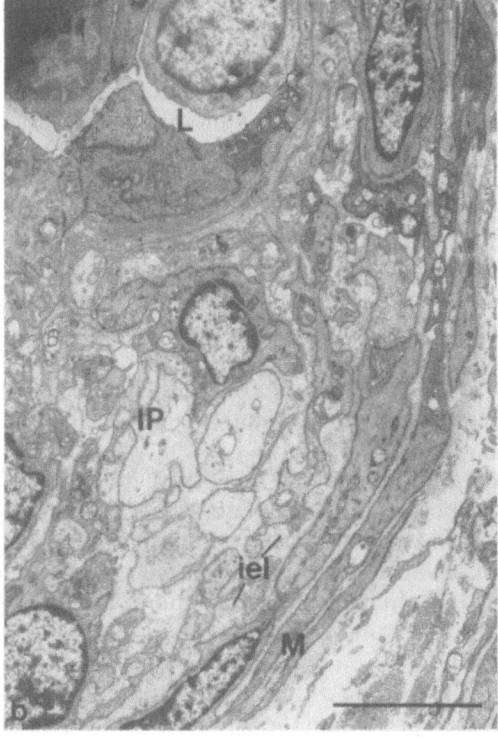

b

Fig. 3a. Photomicrograph of pulmonary hypertensive lung stained for alpha actin isotype showing a marked reduction in immunostaining of the inner part of the media, indicating less differentiated smooth muscle cells in the absence of intimal proliferation.

Fig. 3b. Electromicrograph of peripheral pulmonary artery showing intimal proliferation (IP) composed of relatively undifferentiated smooth muscle cells lying within an internal elastic lamina (iel) and an arc of medial smooth muscle cells (M). L = lumen.

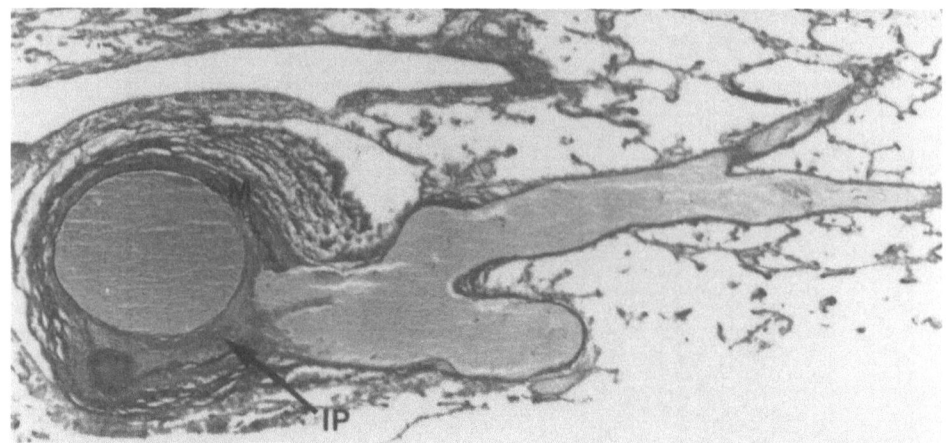

Fig. 4. Photomicrograph of autopsy lung tissue obtained from a 5-month-old child with TGA with VSD (pulmonary vascular resistance = 14 units m^2). A terminal bronchiolar artery distended by injection medium having a thick media (M) and lying internal to the internal elastic lamina intimal proliferation (IP) surrounds the origin of thin-walled branches. (Millers elastic stain counterstained with van Gieson's stain).

and collagen, particularly type-I collagen is deposited in the media and forms the bulk of an expanding adventitia. In the normal baby the pulmonary vascular smooth muscle cells are immature at birth, containing predominantly synthetic rather than contractile myofilaments, and the proportion of contractile myofilaments increases gradually during the first year of life [3, 4]. In pulmonary hypertensive babies however, the formation of contractile myofilaments is accelerated such that the myofilament concentration normally achieved by 6 months of life is seen during the first week of life [7]. The smooth cells of the inner media, those closest to the endothelium, remain relatively differentiated, contain fewer myofilaments and appear to contain less actin (Fig. 3). It is from these cells that intimal proliferation originates. Exuberant cellular intimal proliferation develops rapidly in the walls of all arteries as they enter the respiratory unit (Fig. 4) [8]. The obstruction to flow is strategically placed to increase resistance to flow in all pathways throughout the lung (Fig. 5). Intimal proliferation is seen from 2 months of age and is abundant by 5 months [9]. As the intimal obstruction increases in severity, so the muscularity decreases in more distal vessels (Fig. 6). After 7—9 months of age the medial thickness is usually normal, or even less than normal in the distal vessels (Fig. 7). Such patients have a high resistance and are usually inoperable.

In these young children intimal proliferation is severe and obstructive and pulmonary vascular resistance is elevated before there has been sufficient time to develop the marked intimal fibrosis, medial atrophy, elastosis and generalised arterial dilatation which is characteristic of advanced pulmonary vascular disease and an elevated resistance in older patients [10]. In clinical practise there is rarely any need to biopsy the lung to determine the potential reversibility of the pathological lesions in children with TGA and VSD.

For many years the potential reversibility of the different types of pathological lesions was the only factor considered when predicting the outcome of intracardiac

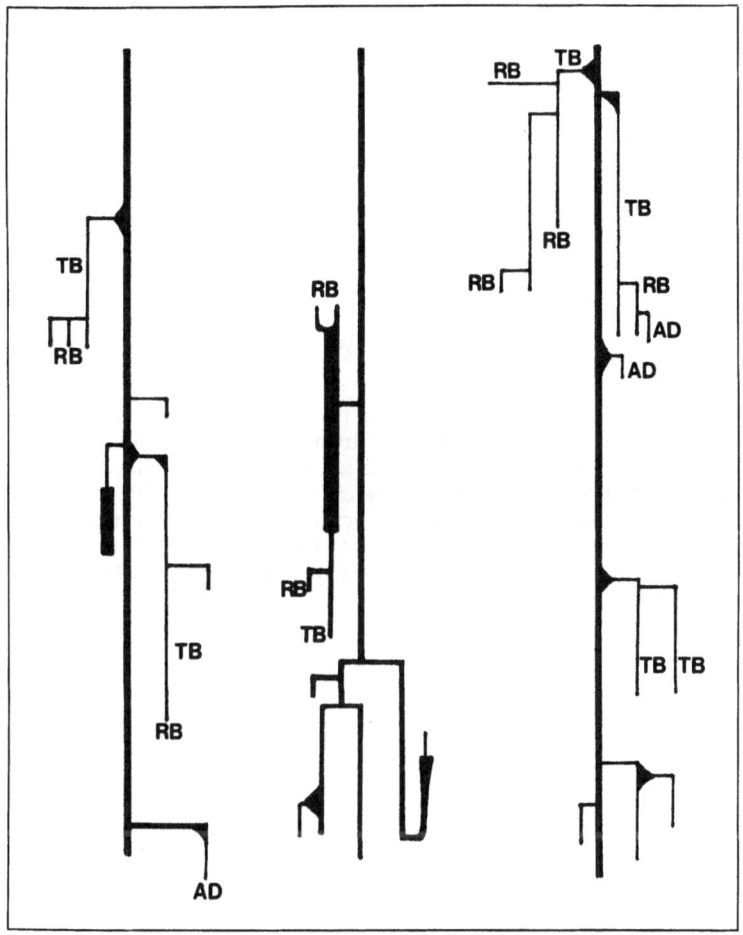

Fig. 5. Diagrams of three pulmonary arterial pathways reconstructed by microscopic serial sectioning. AD, arteries accompanying alveolar ducts; RB, arteries accompanying respiratory bronchioli; TB, arteries accompanying terminal bronchioli.

repair. However, potential reversibility is not synonymous with operability [9]. The patient must first survive the operation. Patients with excessively thick-walled peripheral arteries are prone to develop pulmonary hypertensive crises in the post-operative period (Fig. 8) [11]. These events tend to cluster and can be fatal. Early recognition is vital and post-operative monitoring of the pulmonary arterial pressure is mandatory in children at risk. Treatment consists of hyperoxic hyperventilation with administration of vasodilator drugs such as tolazaline and prostacyclin.

Pulmonary hypertensive crises indicate abnormalities in smooth muscle cell function and probably in endothelial control of smooth muscle cell contractility. In babies with TGA and VSD the pulmonary arterial endothelial cells become morphologically abnormal during the first 6 months of life but endothelial dysfunction can precede morphological injury. For this reason, we investigated the role of cer-

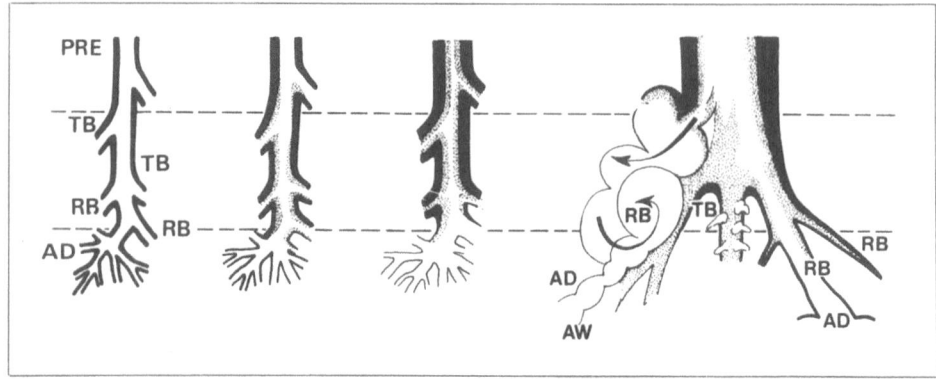

Fig. 6. Diagram of the end of four arterial pathways, from the preacinar (pre-respiratory region, PRE) and terminal bronchiolar arteries (TB) to the intra-acinar (within respiratory region) respiratory bronchiolar (RB) and alveolar duct (AD) arteries, showing the gradual development of intimal proliferation (stippling) associated with the progressive increase in wall thickness of pre-acinar arteries and decrease in wall thickness of intra-acinar arteries until dilatation lesions develop. The upper interrupted line indicates the plane of section of satisfactory biopsies and the lower line is the plane of section of biopsies taken too close to the pleura to sample the distal pre-acinar and all the intra-acinar vessels.

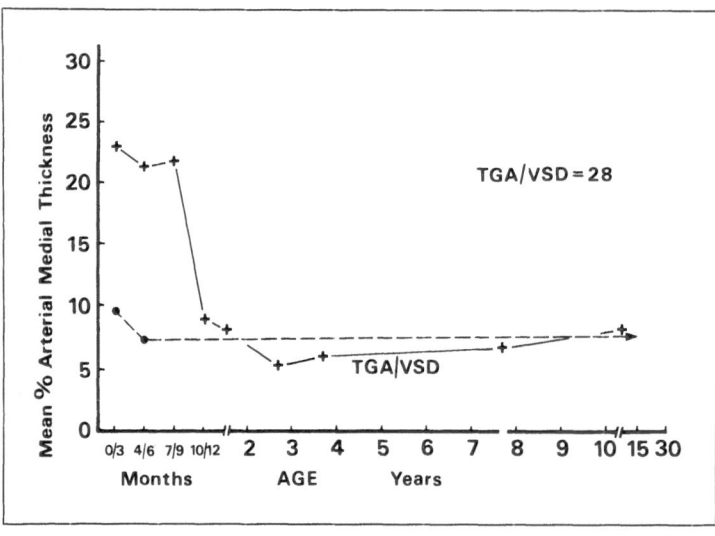

Fig. 7. Percentage pulmonary arterial thickness in arteries 50–100 μm in diameter, related to age in lung biopsies from 28 children with TGA and VSD. Interrupted line indicates the normal relationship.

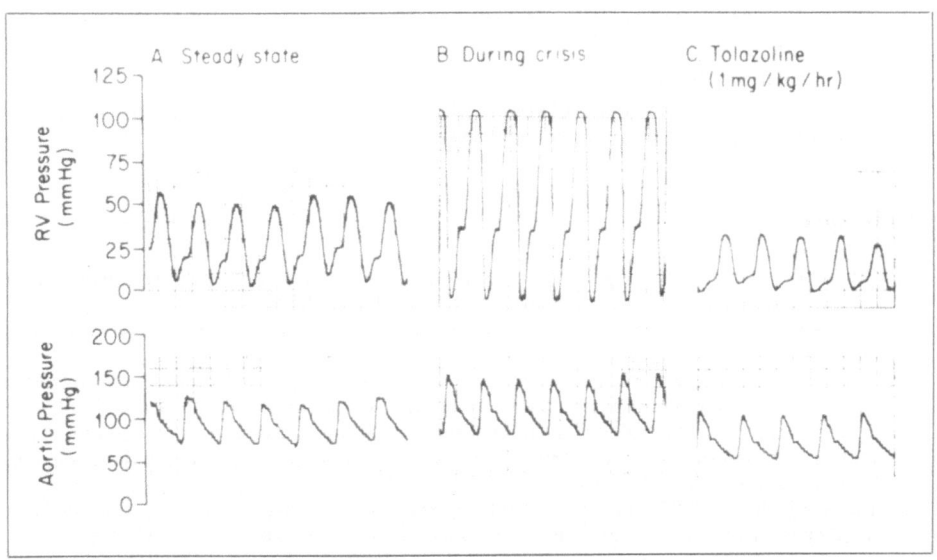

Fig. 8. Pulmonary hypertensive crisis showing a satisfactory response to infusion of tolazoline.

tain vasoactive mediators acting on the vessel wall, and, in some instances, produced by the vessel wall itself. Endothelin is the most potent vasoconstrictor agent yet recognised but we found normal levels of circulating endothelin in our pulmonary hypertensive patients, at all ages, and similar levels of endothelin in the pulmonary arterial and left atrial blood [2]. Despite the presence of a normal circulating level of endothelin however, this peptide may have an important effect at a local cellular level. Also, a normal circulating level of endothelin may be inappropriate in the presence of a diseased pulmonary vascular bed. Eicosanoid biosynthesis was shown to be abnormal in pulmonary hypertensive patients. Prostacyclin has vasodilator and antiplatelet aggregatory actions, while thromboxane B_2 is a vasoconstrictor and proaggregatory substance. We found an imbalance in eicosanoid biosynthesis in favour of thromboxane B_2 in older patients with advanced irreversible pulmonary vascular disease and, also, in young patients with potentially reversible disease [1].

Patients with irreversible pulmonary vascular disease can be helped by a palliative Mustard or Senning procedure which increases systemic arterial oxygen saturation and improves the quality of life [15, 19]. But it does not alter the natural history. Administration of oxygen at night can be beneficial and may perhaps prolong life [5]. The effect of chronic vasodilator therapy is difficult to assess because these drugs also affect the systemic circulation; a favourable response to the acute administration of a vasodilator drug at cardiac catheterisation does not accurately predict the long-term response, and few patients have been subjected to a further cardiac catheterisation study to evaluate the long-term effect of drug administration. Ultimately, the only appropriate treatment available for these patients is a heart/lung transplantation. However, the present 5-year actuarial survival for heart/lung transplantation is only 41%, and patients transplanted for pulmonary vascular disease develop obliterative bronchiolitis more readily than do those transplanted for parenchymal lung disease [12].

In conclusion, pulmonary vascular disease remains the greatest problem in the management of children with TGA and VSD and learning how to control the progression of the disease is a major challenge.

References

1. Adatia IT, Haworth SG (1990) Advanced pulmonary vascular disease: 24 hour urinary excretion of vasoactive eicosanoids. Circulation (Suppl III) 82:A0395
2. Adatia I, Haworth SG (1991) Endothelin in pulmonary hypertensive congenital heart disease. Am Thorac Soc (abstract) 143:A403
3. Allen K, Haworth SG (1988) Human postnatal pulmonary arterial remodelling: ultrastructural studies of smooth muscle cell and connective tissue maturation. Lab Invest 59:702–709
4. Allen K, Haworth SG (1989) Cytoskeletal features of immature pulmonary vascular smooth muscle cells and the influence of pulmonary hypertension on normal human development. J Pathol 158:311–317
5. Bowyer JJ, Busst CM, Denison DM, Shinebourne EA (1986) Effect of long-term oxygen treatment at home in children with pulmonary vascular disease. Br Heart J 55:385–390
6. Ferencz C (1966) Transposition of the great vessels. Pathophysiologic considerations based upon a study of the lungs. Circulation 33:232–241
7. Hall SM, Haworth SG (1991) Onset and evolution of pulmonary vascular disease in young children: abnormal postnatal remodelling studied in lung biopsies. J Pathol (in press)
8. Haworth SG (1984) Pulmonary vascular disease in different types of congenital heart disease. Implications for interpretation of lung biopsy findings in early childhood. Br Heart J 52:557–571
9. Haworth SG, Radley-Smith R, Yacoub M (1987) Lung biopsy findings in transposition of the great arteries with ventricular septal defect: potentially reversible pulmonary vascular disease is not always synonymous with operability. J Am Coll Cardiol 9:327–333
10. Heath D, Edwards JE (1958) The pathology of hypertensive pulmonary vascular disease. A description of six grades of structural changes in the pulmonary artery with special reference to congenital cardiac septal defect. Circulation 18:533–547
11. Jones ODH, Shore DF, Rigby ML, Leijala M, Scallan J, Shinebourne EA, Lincoln JCR (1981) The use of tolazoline hydrochloride as a pulmonary vasodilator in potentially fatal episodes of pulmonary vasoconstriction after cardiac surgery in children. Circulation 64 (Suppl II):134–139
12. Kriett JM, Kaye MP (1991) The registry of the international society for heart and lung transplantation: Eight offical report. J Heart Lung Transplant 10:491–498
13. Leanage R, Agnetti A, Graham G, Taylor J, Macartney FJ (1981) Factors influencing survival after balloon atrial septostomy for complete transposition of the great arteries. Br Heart J 45:559–572
14. Liebman J, Cullum L, Belloc NB (1969) Natural history of transposition of the great arteries. Anatomy and birth and death characteristics. Circulation 40:237–262
15. Lindesmith GG, Stiles QR, Tucker BL, Gallaher ME, Stanton RE, Meyer BW (1972) The Mustard operation as a palliative procedure. J Thorac Cardiovasc Surg 63:75–80
16. Mustard WT, Keith JD, Trusler GA, Fowler R, Kidd L (1964) The surgical management of transposition of the great vessels. J Thorac Cardiovasc Surg 48:953–958
17. Newfeld EA, Paul MH, Muster AJ, Idriss FS (1974) Pulmonary vascular disease in complete transposition of the great arteries. A study of 200 patients. Am J Cardiol 34:75–82
18. Senning A (1959) Surgical correction of transposition of the great arteries. Surgery 45:966–980
19. Stark J, De Leval M, Macartney F, Taylor J (1980) Surgery for transposition of the great arteries with pulmonary vascular obstructive disease. Pediatr Cardiol 1:241 (abstract)
20. Yacoub MH, Radley-Smith R, Hilton CJ (1976) Anatomical correction of complete transposition of the great arteries and ventricular septal defect in infancy. Br Med J 1:1112–1116

21. Yacoub M, Radley-Smith R, Maclaurin R (1977) Two-stage operation for anatomical correction of transposition of the great arteries with intact ventricular septum (abstract). Br Heart J 39:925
22. Yacoub M, Bernhard A, Lange P, Radley-Smith R, Keck E, Stephan E, Heintzen P (1980) Clinical and hemodynamic results of the two-stage anatomic correction of simple transposition of the great arteries. Circulation 62 (Suppl I):190−196

Author's address:
Dr. S. G. Haworth
Hospital for Sick Children
Greet Ormond Street
London WC1 N3JH, G3

Cineangiographic diagnosis of coronary artery anatomy in transposition of the great arteries and double outlet right ventricle: Significance of aortic intramural coronary arteries
A study of 103 patients undergoing arterial switch operation and 16 neonates with elective Senning-Brom operation

U. Sauer
Pediatric Clinic for Heart and Circulatory Disorders, German Heart Center, Munich, FRG

A brief review of the literature

Bill Rashkind's balloon septostomy [29] dramatically changed the natural history of newborn infants with simple, complete transposition of the great arteries (TGA), as it enabled 90% survival for 30 days or more after birth before definitive repair [15].

In recent years, successful arterial switch repair, either as primary or as two-stage procedure after banding of the pulmonary artery in infants with TGA and intact ventricular septum (IVS), or with ventricular septal defect (VSD) or double outlet right ventricle (DORV) became possible with a low operative mortality (2–10%) and an infrequent incidence of significant complications at midterm follow-up [6–9, 13–15, 17, 18, 20–22, 24, 26–28, 31, 34–36].

However, only if the arterial switch operation in simple TGA is carried out within the first days of life – possibly after the diagnosis has been established during early pregnancy by fetal echocardiography [1, 2] – a balloon septostomy may not be necessary. A further advantage of immediate postnatal repair is that the 10% mortality which may occur during the interval between balloon septostomy and definitive repair may be avoided [15].

Most of the early deaths after the arterial switch operation have been related to the complex coronary artery anatomy and the inherent difficulties of transfer to the neoaorta (native pulmonary artery) [6–9, 17, 21, 24, 26, 36]. Furthermore, recatheterization with aortography has documented in several cases the persisting hazard if silent, asymptomatic occlusion of one major coronary artery branch. In these patients, the gradual onset of stenosis allowed the dependent myocardium to become perfused through collaterals from the unobstructed contralateral artery [7–9, 21].

A particularly high risk was found to be associated with:

1) An inverted origin and course of one or both coronary arteries, e.g., in cases in which both coronary arteries originate from the same aortic sinus or with the left circumflex artery (LCX) running posteriorly of the pulmonary artery (neoaorta), making it liable for stenosis after translocation (Fig. 1);

97

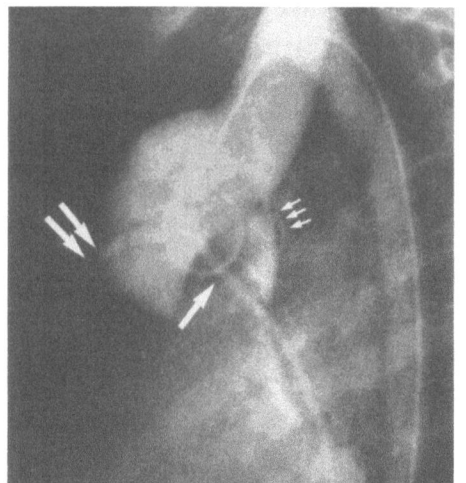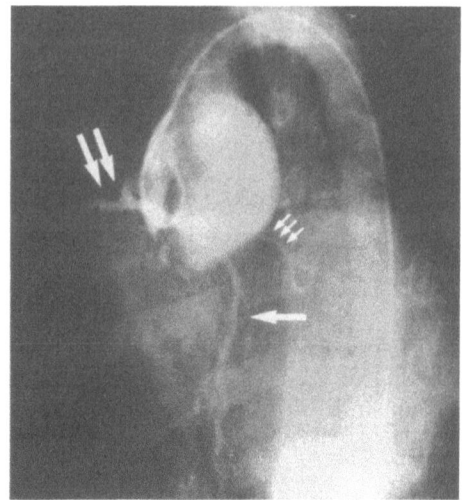

a   b

Fig. 1. 3.8-year-old girl with right side-by-side DORV, i.e., TGA with VSD and aortic orifice slightly right anterior oblique of pulmonary orifice. Type AB II 1 RLAD, 2 CX coronary artery pattern: RCA which gives off LAD from facing sinus 1 and LCX from facing sinus 2 running behind the pulmonary orifice (neoaorta). Aortogram 3.7 years after arterial switch operation and transpulmonary VSD-patch closure. Lateral view (a) and left anterior oblique position, PA view (b): Severe stenosis of proximal LCX (triple arrow), unobstructed RCA (double arrow) and LAD (single arrow). In addition, there was severe LV insufficiency with hypo- and dyskinesia of the antero-lateral wall, severe mitral insufficiency and mild to moderate insufficiency of neoaortic valve.

2) Eccentric location of both ostia directly adjacent to the interostial commissure in association with position of the aortic orifice directly in front of the pulmonary orifice (AP − TGA); and

3) An aortic intramural coronary artery [7−11, 17, 21, 24, 26, 35, 36].

Improved feasibility for the arterial switch operation was achieved by the introduction of several important modifications of the method of transfer of the coronary arteries; these procedures were designed to avoid stretching, kinking, and torsion, as well as injury and compression [4, 7, 8, 17, 21, 22, 26, 28, 35].

Only a few studies have been published in which a preoperative detailed diagnosis of the coronary artery anatomy was established either by echocardiography [25] or angiography [19] which was compared with the intraoperative findings and related to the outcome after arterial switch operation.

In our experience, a perfect arterial switch operation for TGA requires an accurate diagnosis of the coronary artery anatomy as part of the preoperative diagnosis. Up to now, this is best achieved by cineangiography [30].

The aim of this study was to delineate angiographic features of the coronary artery anatomy which would be predictive of problems during the arterial switch operation.

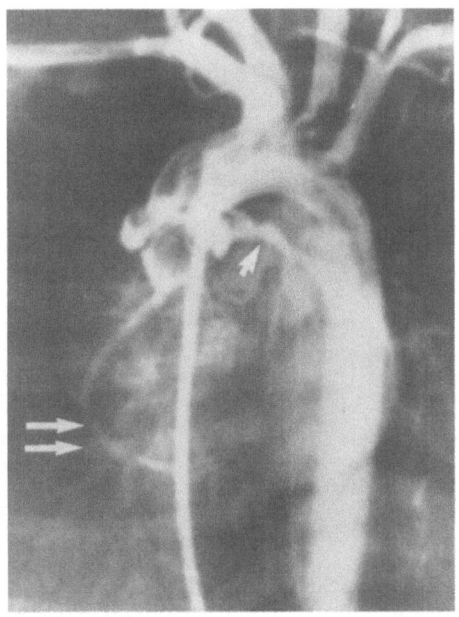

Fig. 2. Aortogram in left anterior oblique position 16°, cranially angled 10°, PA view of newborn girl with D-TGA (aortic orifice right anterior oblique of pulmonary orifice) and intact septum with most common coronary artery pattern, type A I 1L, 2R: LCA (arrow head) from facing sinus 1 and RCA (double arrow) from facing sinus 2.

Patients and methods

Two groups of patients were included in this study:
Group 1 consisted of 103 consecutive patients (72 male and 31 female) with TGA or DORV who underwent an arterial switch operation in our hospital from May 1983 through December 1990. Their ages ranged from 3 days to 13.5 years, median age 13 days: nine patients were <7 days, 51 patients 7–14 days, and 43 patients >15 days.

Group 2 included 16 consecutive neonates, 15 were male and one female, (<30 days old) with TGA in whom an arterial switch operation seemed not feasible and, therefore, a Senning-Brom operation was performed in the calendar year 1990. Two patients were <7 days, 10 patients 7–14 days, and four patients were >15 days. Generally, in the neonates and young infants a Rashkind balloon septostomy was performed during diagnostic catheterization and cineangiography. To demonstrate the coronary arteries, generally, a transvenous antegrade aortogram was performed with the inflated balloon catheter in the ascending aorta in standard posteroanterior (PA) and lateral projections, occasionally with some left or right oblique orientation (Fig. 2). More recently, a complementary "laid-back" caudal view aortogram with balloon occlusion of the ascending aorta was used in some patients [19] (Fig. 3a, b). All preoperative angiograms were reviewed for:

1) the coronary artery anatomy: ostia, branching, and course of coronary arteries; and
2) the spatial relationship of the orifices of the great arteries.

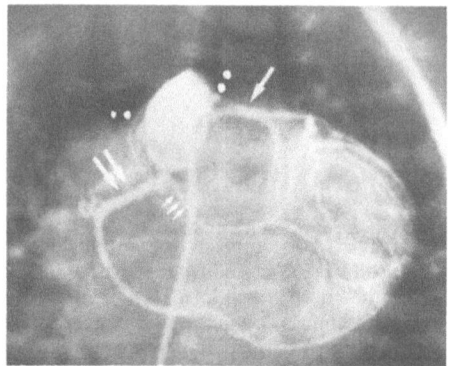
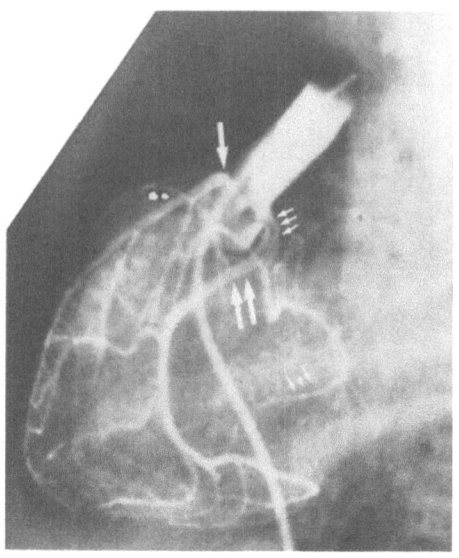

a   b

Fig. 3. Aortogram in laid-back view (a) (with frontal camera caudally angled 30°) and lateral view (b) of male neonate with D-TGA and intact septum with second most common coronary artery pattern, type ABI 1LAD, 2CXR: LAD (single arrow) giving off a conal branch (double dot) from facing sinus 1, RCA (double arrow) which gives off LCX (triple arrow) from facing sinus 2.

The interrelationship between the infundibular septum, aligned and malaligned VSD, spatial relationship between aorta and pulmonary artery, and the coronary artery pattern had been documented previously [10, 16, 33].

In addition, all operative reports were reviewed. Follow-up information on the current clinical status of the surviving patients and the causes of death were based on the review of the hospital records and autopsy findings if available.

Group 1 with arterial switch operation, anatomy, operative management and follow-up

The prevalence of VSD, DORV, and bicuspid pulmonary valve (neoaorta) is shown in Table 1. The DORV was of the Taussig-Bing variety in 10 patients. In two patients, one with a VSD and the other with DORV, the ventricles were in superior/inferior position. Eighty-three patients had a primary switch operation

Table 1. DHM Arterial switch operation (103 patients)

	TGA-IVS	TGA-VSD	DORV
	59(4+)	30(5+)	14(1+)
COA	1	6	4
PAV bi	0	2	2

deaths: intra-op n = 4; hospital n = 3; late n = 3

100

and 20 patients had a two-stage switch repair after previous pulmonary artery banding with concurrent resection of a coarctation in four patients, enlargement of an atrial septal defect (ASD) in three patients, and an aorto-pulmonary shunt in an 8-month-old boy with TGA, restrictive VSD, and severely impaired right ventricular (RV) function. At definitive arterial switch repair, an ASD was closed with a patch in 63 patients; 50 of these patients had a previous balloon septostomy. The VSD was closed with a patch in 35 patients, including all patients with DORV, by direct suture in eight patients and it was left open in one. There were seven hospital deaths and three late deaths (7 months; 1.0 and 3.3 years postoperative). The intraoperative death in three of four infants was primarily related to coronary artery complications, and due to a combination of problems in one infant with associated coarctation, which had been missed preoperatively, and injury of a coronary artery branch. Follow-up information was obtained for 90 of the 93 survivors, with the longest follow-up (until October 1991) being 8.4 years.

Spatial relationship of aorta and pulmonary artery

The angiographic spatial relationship between the orifices of the great arteries and prevalence of VSD and DORV in group 1 is shown in Fig. 4. Each of the three common spatial relationships: Right anterior oblique or D-TGA, anteroposterior or AP-TGA, and left anterior oblique or L-TGA were equally frequently associated with IVS and VSD or DORV. All three patients with a right side-by-side position of the aorta and pulmonary artery also had a VSD, i.e., DORV.

Angiographic coronary artery anatomy

According to the origin from the facing aortic sinuses 1 and 2, and depending on the course of the major coronary arteries, five coronary artery patterns were distinguished in group 1 (Fig. 5) [10, 11, 30]. Seventy-two patients had the usual pattern A I 1 L, 2 R in which the origin and the course of both LCA (L) and RCA (R) were transposed in comparison to the normal situation. All of the remaining 31 patients had either a less common type (AB I 1 LAD, 2 CXR) or rarer types (B I 1 acc AD, 2 LR; B II 1 R, 2 L; AB II 1 RLAD, 2 CX), in which one or both main coronary

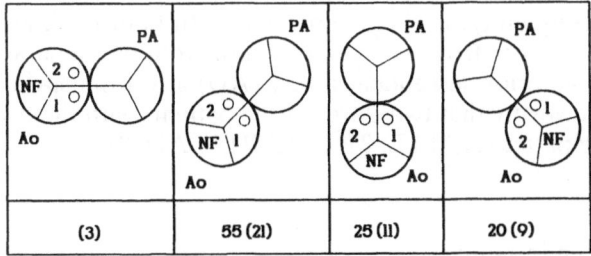

| (3) | 55 (21) | 25 (11) | 20 (9) |

( ) - TGA + VSD or DORV

Fig. 4. Position of aorta and pulmonary artery in 103 patients with TGA ± VSD or DORV and "switch"

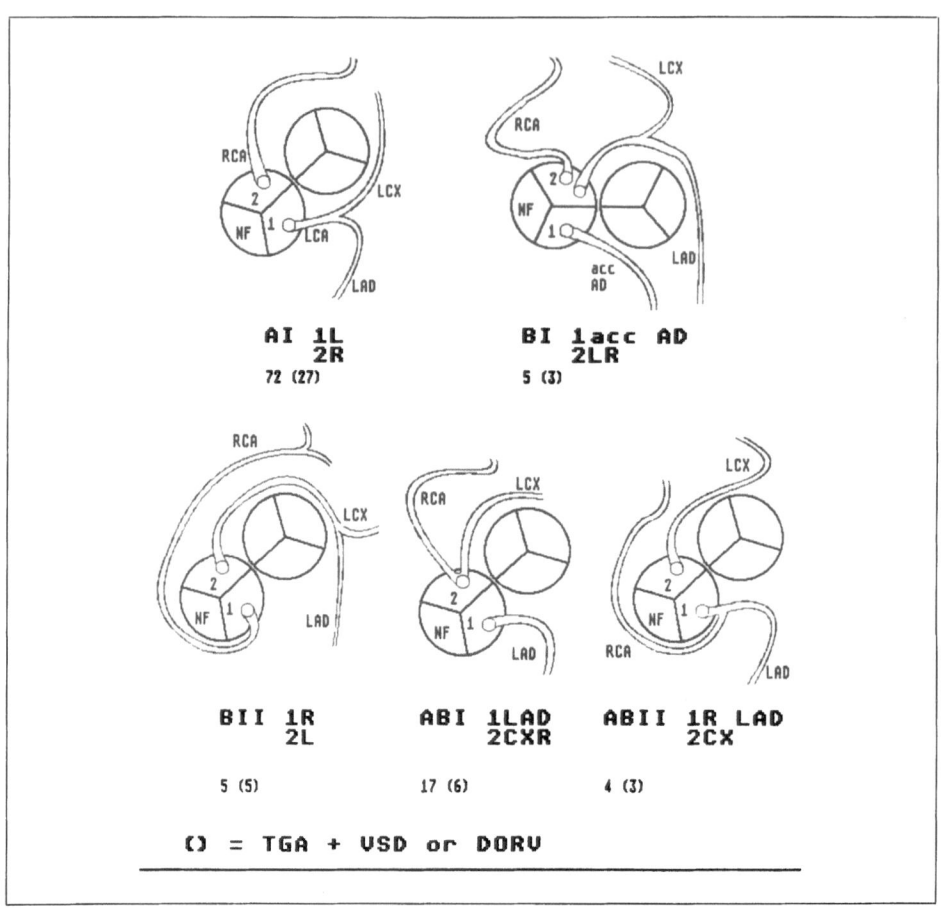

Fig. 5. DHM coronary artery pattern in 103 patients with TGA ± VSD or DORV and arterial switch operation

arteries or the left circumflex artery (CX) in cases with a split LCA were inverted, i.e., not transposed in contrast to the usual pattern in TGA. Accordingly, the course of the LCA was posterior to the pulmonary artery in 10 patients; in nine patients the RCA ran anterior to the aorta, and in 21 patients the LCX ran behind the pulmonary valve. Not infrequently, in the five patients with both LCA and RCA originating from sinus 2, either from a single ostium or from two separate ostia, there was an accessory anterior descendens artery (AD) also from sinus 1 (BI1 acc AD, 2LR). It is noteworthy that two-thirds of the patients with the two most common coronary artery patterns (AI 1L, 2R and ABI 1LAD, 2CXR) also had D-TGA and IVS.

Comparison of preoperative and intraoperative findings

When comparing the preoperative angiographic diagnoses with respect to origin, branching and course of coronary arteries with the intraoperative findings, there

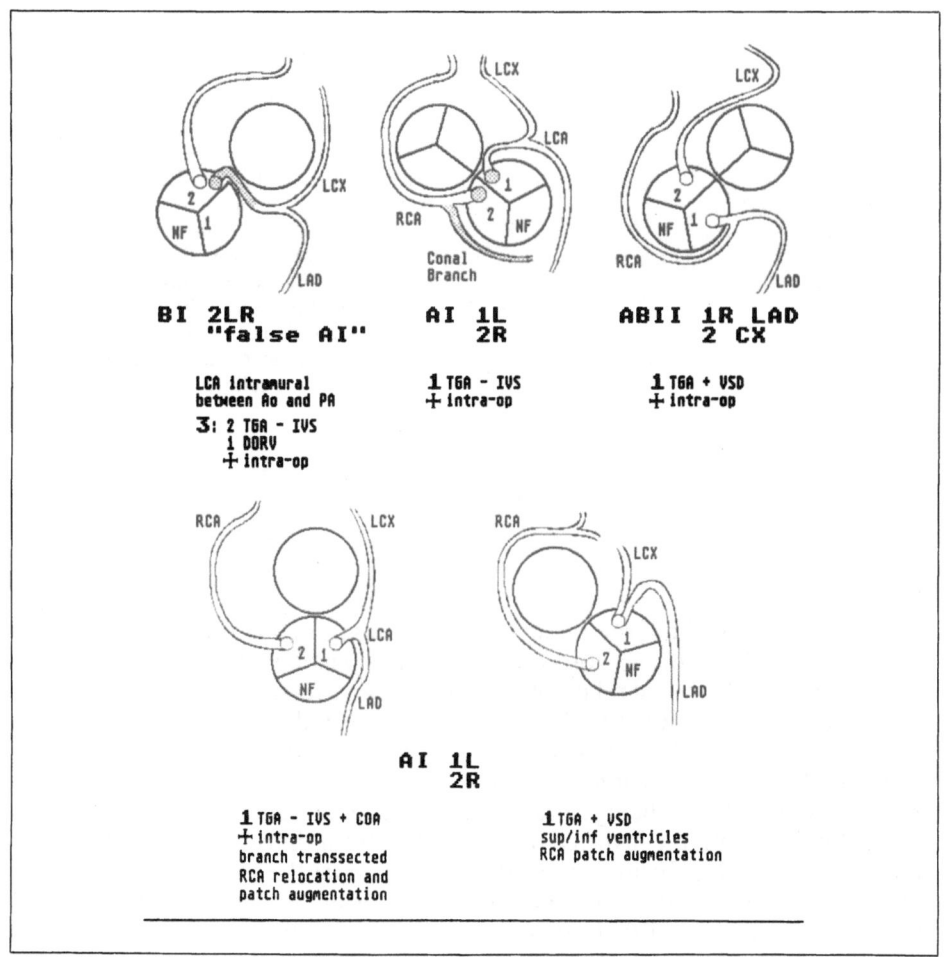

Fig. 6. DHM complications related to coronary arteries in 7 of 103 patients with "switch"

was good correlation in 100 of the 103 patients with switch operation (group 1). On the other hand, surgery added some important anatomical details which had not been demonstrated by preoperative standard aortograms: Two separate ostia in one facing aortic sinus in four children, eccentric location of one or both ostia close to the interostial commissure in six children. Furthermore, in some children at surgery the interostial aortic and pulmonary commissures were not aligned and, therefore, facing of the sinuses was incomplete.

Complications

Complications which were primarily related to the coronary arteries and which had not been suspected on preoperative angiography, in most instances, occurred in seven infants during switch operation (group 1) (Fig. 6). In three patients the prob-

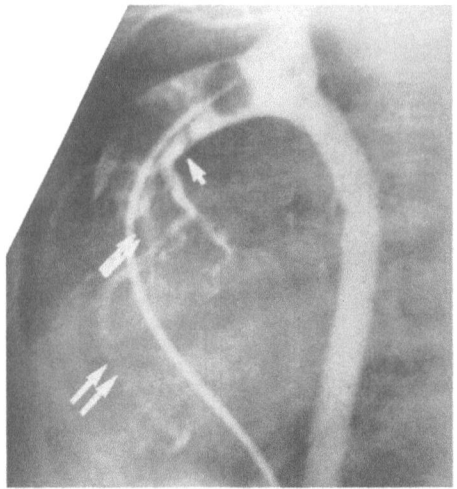

Fig. 7. Three month-old female with DORV and aortic orifice left anterior oblique of pulmonary orifice, with bicuspid pulmonary valve. Preoperative aortogram in lateral view. RCA (double arrow) arises normally from facing sinus 2, while take-off of LCA (arrow head) is high ectopic (B I 2 LR). Initially this was not recognized and an intramural course of LCA between aorta and pulmonary artery was not suspected. False preoperative diagnosis of A I 1 L, 2 R was made. Despite of this, arterial-switch operation was carried out successfully with implantation of LCA high above neoaortic valve and pericard augmentation of left pulmonary artery to relieve compression of LCA.

lems could be resolved surgically, but four infants died intraoperatively. As indicated in Fig. 6, in the three patients who had the usual coronary artery pattern (AI 1 L, 2 R) difficulties in coronary artery translocation seemed to be mainly due to the unfavorable spatial relationship of the great arteries (AP- or L-TGA), combined with close vicinity of both ostia to the interostial commissure in one infant. Type AB II 1 R LAD, 2 CX was angiographically diagnosed at preoperative study, thus indicating the inherent risk because of the inverted tangential origin of RCA from sinus 1, that being a branch of LAD coursing anterior to the aortic valve in combination with the inverted origin of LCX from sinus 2 and its course behind the pulmonary valve. In none of the three patients was the aortic intramural course of the LCA between the aorta and pulmonary artery diagnosed on preoperative angiography (Figs. 7–10). In contrast to the schematic drawing, the aorta was directly in front of the pulmonary artery (AP-TGA) in all three patients, with only a slight leftward deviation in the girl with DORV.

Group 2 with Senning-Brom operation (Table 2)

All patients with Senning-Brom operation had complete TGA with small perimembranous VSD in two. A balloon septostomy was performed at diagnostic catheterization in all patients. The primary contraindication against an arterial switch operation was the complex coronary artery anatomy in 10 patients: AB I 1 LAD, 2 CXR in five patients, AB II 1 R LAD, 2 CX (Fig. 11), B II 1 R, 2 L with both coronary arteries being inverted, B I with single right coronary artery from sinus 2 with only an accessory anterior descending artery from sinus 1 and an intramural LCA in B I-like pattern and an intramural RCA in A II-like pattern, each in one patient, respectively. Additional contraindications were: low systolic pressure in LV, anatomical rather than functional LV outflow tract obstruction, significant difference between aortic and pulmonary valve size and great distance between LCA and neoaorta in association with an unfavorable great arterial relationship.

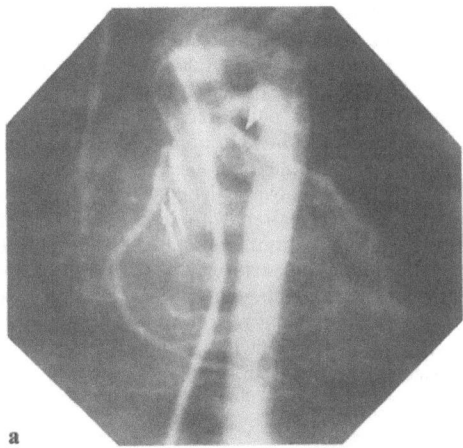

a

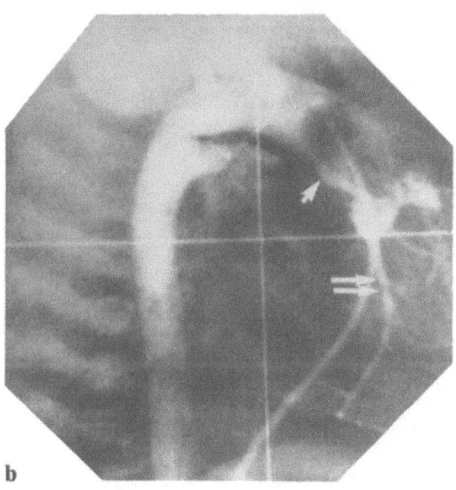

b

Fig. 8. Preoperative aortogram of 3-day-old male neonate with anteroposterior AP-TGA, i.e., aortic orifice slightly left anterior oblique of pulmonary orifice, with intact septum and B I 2LR coronary artery pattern. PA view (a) mimics, however, the most common type A I 1L, 2R with LCA (arrow head) from facing sinus 1 and RCA (double arrow) from facing sinus 2. Only on lateral view (b) the ectopic high origin of LCA is recognized with minimal bulging of right aortic wall as it runs leftward across aorta to reach the anterior interventricular groove. These findings were initially missed and intramural course between aorta and pulmonary artery was not suspected. During arterial-switch operation (at 10 days), the anatomical problem was resolved by implanting RCA and LCA high above neoaortic sinuses and pericard augmentation of pulmonary trunk which had caused compression of the newly implanted LCA resulting in LV dilatation and pulmonary edema.

The causes of postoperative death in the two infants were cerebral bleeding and septicemia. Short-term follow-up in the 14 surviving children is maximally 2.1 years.

Aortic intramural coronary arteries: Own cases and cases from 6 publications

The incidence of an intramural coronary artery in our total study population was 4% (5 of 119): three in the Switch-Group 1 (Figs. 7–10) and two in the Senning-Group 2. In our own cases and in the cases from the literature, an intramural coronary artery was found basically in three types of coronary artery pattern (Fig. 12):

1) With all main coronary artery branches from sinus 2 (B I 2LR, e.g., Shaher's Fig. 5a in [32], Gittenberger-de Groot's Figs. 1 and 2 in [11], and Mayer's "intramural LCA and LAD" in [21];

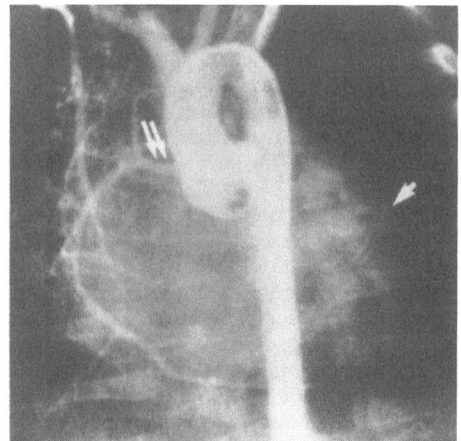

Fig. 9. Same patient as in Fig. 8. At recatheterization 2 months after arterial switch operation, the aortogram in PA (a) and lateral views (b and c) shows only retrograde filling of LCA (white arrow) through collaterals from dilated RCA (double arrow) in right dominant coronary circulation which suggests occlusion of proximal LCA at anastomosis with neoaorta. LV function was mildly impaired with inhomogenous wall motion. In addition, there was severe stenosis of right pulmonary artery with almost exclusive perfusion of left lung, hypertension and increased arteriolar resistance in left pulmonary artery concurrent with RV insufficiency and tricuspid regurgitation.

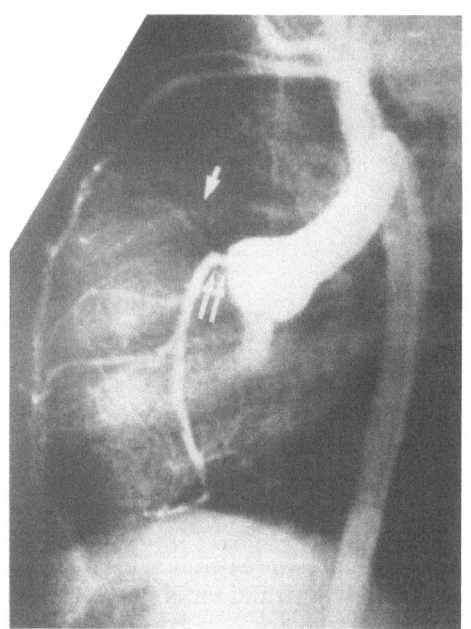

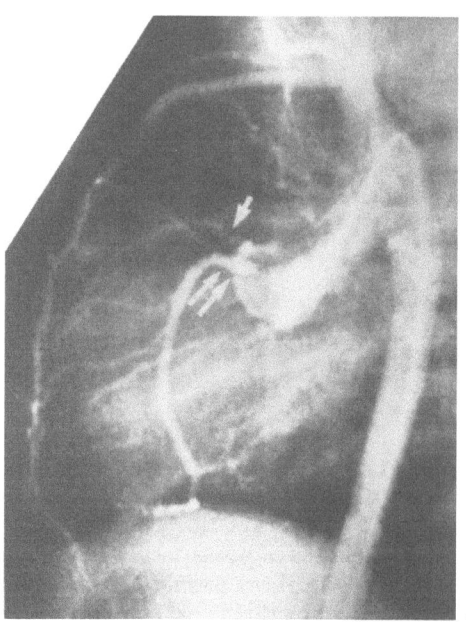

2) With both coronary arteries from sinus 1 (A II 1LR, e.g., Yacoub's type B in [25]; and
3) With inverted RCA and LCA (B II 1R, 2L, e.g., Norwood's case in [24].

In Fig. 12 the cases were categorized according to the anomalous artery: An intramural LCA with course between aorta and pulmonary artery was most common and occurred almost exclusively with type B I 2LR and AP- or D-TGA. Four out of 10 own patients in both surgical groups with the definite intraoperative diagnosis of B I 2 LR had an intramural LCA. On outward inspection [11] and angio-

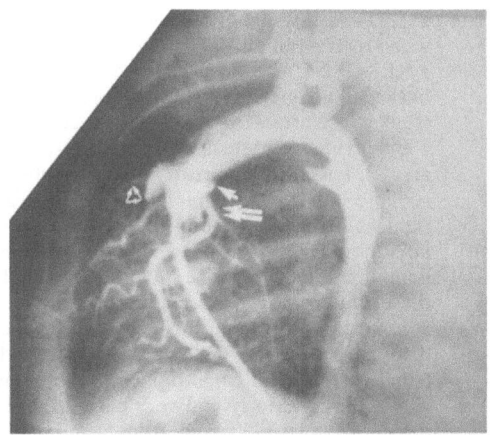

Fig. 10. Male neonate with D-TGA, small VSD and PDA. Preoperative aortogram (lateral view) reveals high ectopic origin of LCA (arrow head) above facing sinus 2 which suspects intramural course of LCA between the aorta and pulmonary artery. RCA (double arrow) arises from facing sinus 2 (BI 2LR). Accessory anterior descending artery from facing sinus 1 (open triangle). Initially, A I 1 L, 2 R was falsely diagnosed. During arterial switch operation (at 11 days), on external inspection the intramural course of LCA could not be recognized and the artery was transected during mobilization of ostium. Therefore, arterial switch operation was aborted in favor of Senning-operation, but the patient died in tabula.

Table 2. Senning-operation instead of arterial switch operation in 16 neonates with TGA ± VSD (1. 1. 1988–31. 12. 1990): Coronary artery pattern and associated position of orifices of aorta and pulmonary artery, preoperative or intraoperative decision against arterial switch operation and outcome

Coronary artery pattern	n	Orifices of great arteries			IVS	VSD	Decision		Lived	Died
		right oblique D	left oblique L	antero- post. AP			preop.	intraop.		inhosp.
AI1L,2R	6	1	1	4	4	2	2	4	5	1
ABI1LAD,2CXR	5	4	1	–	5	–	2	3	5	–
BI2LR	1	1	–	–	1	–	–	1	1	–
LCA intramural	1	–	–	1	–	1	1	–	1	–
AII1LR RCA intramural	1	1	–	–	1	–	1	–	–	1
BII1R,2L	1	1	–	–	1	–	–	1	1	–
ABII1RLAD,2CX	1	1	–	–	1	–	1	–	1	–

L, LCA, left coronary artery; R, RCA, right coronary artery; CX, LCX, left circumflex artery; LAD, left anterior descending artery; IVS, intact ventricular septum

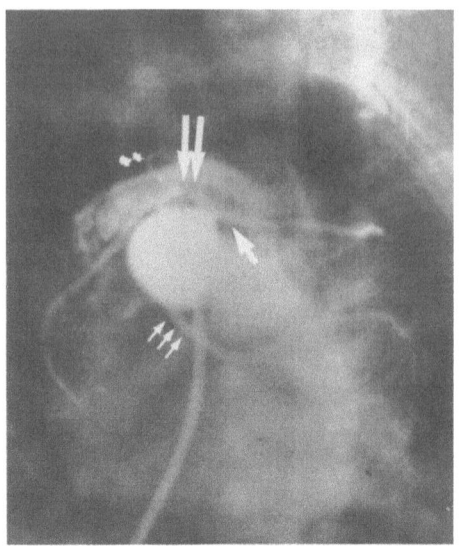

Fig. 11. Aortogram of 3-day-old male neonate with D-TGA, small VSD and PDA with AB II 1 RLAD, 2 CX coronary artery pattern. Laid-back caudal view (a) shows short common trunk which arises from mid of left facing sinus 1 and divides at acute angle into RCA (double arrow), LAD (single arrow) and conal branch (double dot). LCX (triple arrow) arises from right facing sinus 2 and gives rise to postero-lateral branches and sinus node artery running behind pulmonary orifice. On lateral view (b) these findings are confirmed: Short common coronary artery trunk from facing sinus 1 which trifurcates into RCA (double arrow), LAD (single arrow) and conal branch (double dot) which run anteriorly and very close to aortic orifice, LCX (triple arrow) from facing sinus 2 coursing behind pulmonary orifice. Because of risk for tension of RCA and kinking of LAD on transfer into neoaorta, arterial switch operation was aborted in favor of Senning-operation.

a

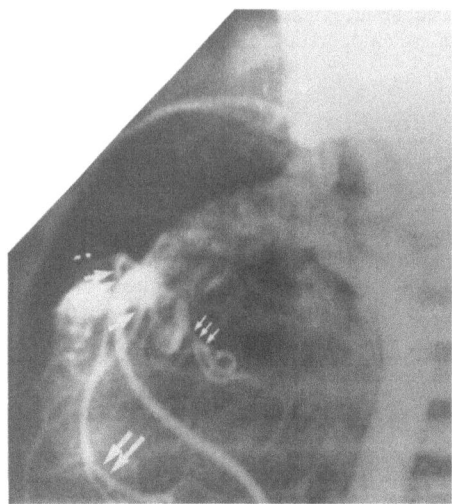

b

graphy (Fig. 8), it can mimic the common type A I 1 L, 2 R coronary pattern. A total of 13 patients with this anatomy underwent an arterial switch operation with nine survivors and four deaths [6, 9, 21, 24, 26, 36].

As in Norwood's case [24], occassionally in type B II 1 R, 2 L, the LCA can run intramurally, giving the false appearance of type A II 1 LR. The second most common intramural artery was the RCA. Since it occurred always in association with type A II 1 LR (Yacoub's type B [35]), it can mimic "false A I 1 L, 2 R". Of special interest were the cases with B I 2 LR, in which sinus 2 gave rise to all main coronary arteries from separate ostia. Regularly, one ostium was eccentric and close to the interostial commissure, giving rise to an intramural artery: RCA together with

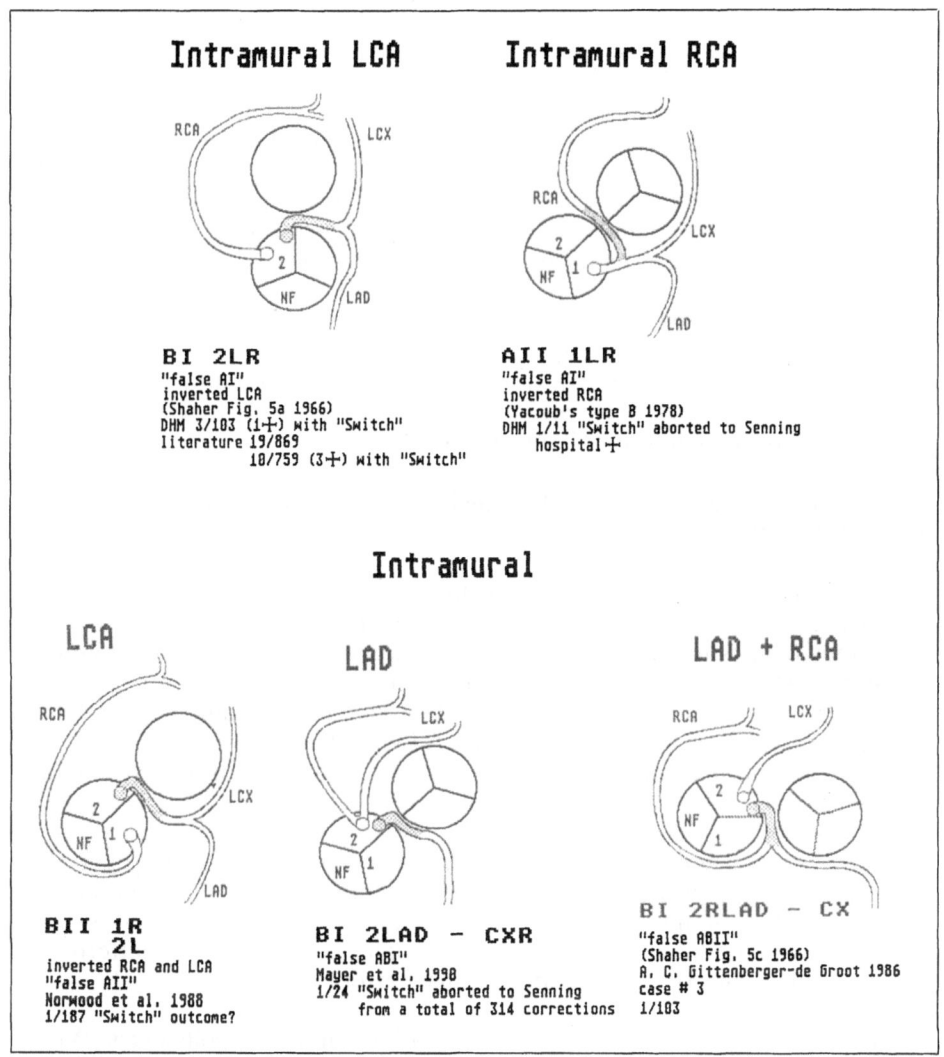

Fig. 12. ■

LAD (B I 2 R LAD − CX) can mimic "false AB II 1 R LAD, 2 CX" [11, 32], or the individual LAD (B I 2 LAD − CXR) falsely suggested AB I (1 LAD 2 CXR) [21].

Conclusion

This study confirms that the coronary artery anatomy in the neonate with TGA and DORV and variable spatial relationship of the great arteries can be accurately diagnosed by antegrade aortography in standard and/or "laid-back" views. Additional information on the number and location of the ostia within the aortic sinuses in relation to the commissures, alignment of the interostial commissures and completeness of facing of aortic and pulmonary sinuses should be obtained from complementary echocardiography. Our experience further attests that all coronary artery patterns are "switchable" in the neonate with simple complete TGA, or older infant with TGA and large VSD or DORV, all with good midterm results. We submit, in consistency with the experience of others, that complications during arterial switch operation relate to the complex coronary anatomy primarily if associated with an inverted, not transposed origin and course which is commonly associated with uncommon spatial relationship of the great arteries. Two other pathologic entities which significantly increase operative risk are:

1) Eccentric ostia close to the interostial commissure with tangential take-off of the coronary artery, and
2) Ectopic high take-off or eccentric ostium of an aortic intramural coronary artery with course between aorta and pulmonary artery which are either in anteroposterior or right anterior oblique position.

Thus, features which at preoperative angiography can predict an intramural coronary artery are:

1) One facing sinus without coronary ostium;
2) All main coronary artery branches from the other facing sinus;
3) Ostium of intramural (inverted) coronary artery is generally eccentric and close to interostial commissure or ectopic above it;
4) LCA is most commonly involved, RCA second most commonly, rarely RCA together with LAD or LAD alone, never LCX (thus far);
5) The intramural coronary artery always runs between aorta and pulmonary artery.

If in patients with aortic intramural coronary artery an arterial switch operation is aborted in favor of the Senning-operation, the hazard of sudden death remains [3, 5, 11, 12, 23]. Attempts to extend the indication for an arterial switch operation with the use of modified techniques to all complex coronary artery patterns, with the inclusion of the aortic intramural coronary arteries will be beneficial.

Acknowledgements: I wish to express my gratitude to all my colleagues. Without their expert diagnosis, surgical and medical treatment, and dedicated care of our patients this study would not have been possible.

I am also particularly grateful to Misses Yvonne Aeschbach and Michaela Maier for their assistance in the preparation of the manuscript, to Mrs. Ingeborg Klein and Mrs. Brigitte Hedrich for their secretarial work, to Dr. med. Th. Genz for computer design work, and to Mrs. Helena Soik for photography.

References

1. Allan LD, Tynan MJ, Campbell S, Wilkinson JL, Anderson RH (1980) Echocardiographic and anatomical correlates in the fetus. Br Heart J 44:445–451
2. Allan LD, Chita SK, Sharland G, Fagg N, Anderson RH, Crawford DC (1989) The accuracy of fetal echocardiography in the diagnosis of congenital heart disease. Int J Cardiol 25:279–288

3. Angelini P (1989) Normal and anomalous coronary arteries: Definition and classification. Am Heart J 117:418−434
4. Aubert J, Pannetier A, Couvelly JP, Unal D, Rounault F, Delarue A (1978) Transposition of the great arteries: New technique for anatomical correction. Br Heart J 40:204−208
5. Barth III CW, Bray M, Roberts WC (1986) Sudden death in infancy associated with origin of both left main and right coronary arteries from a common ostium above the left sinus of Valsalva. Am J Cardiol 57:365−366
6. Brawn WJ, Mee RBB (1988) Early results for anatomic correction of transposition of the great arteries and for double-outlet right ventricle with subpulmonary ventricular septal defect. J Thorac Cardiovasc Surg 95:230−238
7. Castaneda AR, Norwood WJ, Jonas RA, Colan SD, Sanders SP, Lang P (1984) Transposition of the great arteries and intact ventricular septum: Anatomical repair in the neonate. Ann Thorac Surg 38:438−443
8. Castaneda AR, Trusler GA, Paul MH, Blackstone EH, Kirklin JW, Congenital Heart Surgeons Society (1988) The early results of treatment of simple transposition in the current era. J Thorac Cardiosvasc Surg 95:14−28
9. Di Donato RM, Wernovsky G, Walsh EP, Colan SD, Lang P, Wessel DL, Jonas RA, Mayer JE, Castaneda AR (1989) Results of the arterial switch operation for transposition of the great arteries with ventricular septal defect. Surgical considerations and midterm follow-up data. Circulation 80:1689−1705
10. Gittenberger-de Groot AC, Sauer U, Oppenheimer-Dekker A, Quaegebeur JM (1983) Coronary arterial anatomy in transposition of the great arteries: A morphologic study. Pediatr Cardiol 4 (Suppl I):15−24
11. Gittenberger-de Groot AC, Sauer U, Quaegebeur JM (1986) Aortic intramural coronary artery in three hearts with transposition of the great arteries. J Thorac Cardiovasc Surg 91:566−571
12. Imamura T, Nakagawa S, Koiwaya Y, Tanaka K, Saisho K, Sumiyoshi A (1986) Recurrent myocardial infarction and unexpected sudden death in a case of d-loop d-transposition of the great arteries associated with single coronary artery. Clin Cardiol 9:77−81
13. Jatene AD, Fontes VF, Souza LCB, Paulista PP, Abdulmassih Neto C, Sousa JEMR, Zerbini EJ (1982) Anatomic correction of transposition of the great arteries. J Thorac Cardiovasc Surg 83:20−26
14. Jonas RA (1991) Update on the rapid two-stage arterial switch procedure. Cardiology in the Young 1:99−100
15. Kirklin JW (1991) The surgical repair for complete transposition. Cardiology in the Young 1:13−25
16. Kurosawa H, Imai Y, Takanashi Y, Hoshino S, Sawatari K, Kawada M, Takao A (1986) Infundibular septum and coronary anatomy in Jatene operation. J Thorac Cardiovasc Surg 91:572−583
17. Kurosawa H, Imai Y, Kawada M (1991) Coronary arterial anatomy in regard to the arterial switch procedure. Cardiology in the Young 1:54−62
18. Losay J, Planché C, Gerardin B, Lacour-Gayet F, Bruniaux J, Kachaner J (1990) Midterm surgical results of arterial switch operation for transposition of the great arteries with intact septum. Circulation 82 (Suppl IV):IV-146−IV-150
19. Mandell VS, Lock JE, Mayer JE, Parness IA, Kulik TJ (1990) The "laid-back" aortogram: An improved angiographic view for demonstration of coronary arteries in transposition of the great arteries. Am J Cardiol 65:1379−1383
20. Mayer JE Jr, Jonas RA, Castaneda AR (1986) Arterial switch operation for transposition of the great arteries with intact ventricular septum. J Cardiac Surg 1:97−104
21. Mayer JE Jr, Sanders SP, Jonas RA, Castaneda AR, Wernovsky G (1990) Coronary artery pattern and outcome of arterial switch operation for transposition of the great arteries. Circulation 82 (Suppl IV):IV-139−IV-145
22. Mee RBB (1991) Results of the arterial switch procedure for complete transposition with an intact ventricular septum. Cardiology in the Young 1:97−98
23. Mustafa J, Gula G, Radley-Smith R, Dürrer S, Yacoub M (1981) Anomalous origin of the left coronary artery from the anterior aortic sinus. A potential cause of sudden death. J Thorac Cardiovasc Surg 82:297−300

24. Norwood WI, Dobell AR, Freed MD, Kirklin JW, Blackstone EH, and the Congenital Heart Surgeons Society (1988) Intermediate results of the arterial switch repair. A 20-institution study. J Thorac Cardiovasc Surg 96:854–863

25. Pasquini L, Sanders SP, Parness IA, Colan SD (1987) Diagnosis of coronary artery anatomy by two-dimensional echocardiography in patients with transposition of the great arteries. Circulation 75:557–564

26. Planché C, Bruniaux J, Lacour-Gayet F, Kachaner J, Binet J-P, Sidi D, Villain E (1988) Switch operation for transposition of the great arteries in neonates. A study of 120 patients. J Thorac Cardiovasc Surg 96:354–363

27. Planché C, Serraf A, Lacour-Gayet F, Bruniaux J, Bouchart F (1991) Anatomic correction of complete transposition with ventricular septal defect in neonates: Experience with 42 consecutive cases. Cardiology in the Young 1:101–103

28. Quaegebeur JM, Rohmer J, Ottenkamp J, Buis T, Kirklin JW, Blackstone EH, Brom AG (1986) The arterial switch operation. An eight-year experience. J Thorac Cardiovasc Surg 92:361–384

29. Rashkind WJ, Miller WW (1966) Creation of an atrial septal defect without thoracotomy. A palliative approach to complete transposition of the great arteries. J Am Med Assoc 196:991–992

30. Sauer U, Gittenberger-de Groot AC, Peters DR, Bühlmeyer K (1983) Cineangiography of the coronary arteries in transposition of the great arteries. Ped Cardiol 4 (Suppl 1):25–42

31. Serraf A, Lacour-Gayet F, Bruniaux J, Losay J, Petit J, Planché C (1990) Anatomic repair of Taussig-Bing (TBH). Abstract Circulation 82 (Suppl III):III-194

32. Shaher RM, Puddu GC (1966) Coronary arterial anatomy in complete transposition of the great vessels. Am J Cardiol 17:355–361

33. Van Praagh R, Perez-Trevino C, Lopez-Cuellar M, Baker FW, Zuberbuhler JR, Quero M, Perez VM, Moreno F, van Praagh S (1971) Transposition of the great arteries with posterior aorta, anterior pulmonary artery, subpulmonary conus and fibrous continuity between aortic and atrioventricular valves. Am J Cardiol 28:621–631

34. Wernovsky G, Hougen TJ, Walsh EP, Sholler GF, Colan SD, Sanders SP, Parness IA, Keane JF, Mayer JE Jr, Jonas RA, Castaneda AR, Lang P (1988) Midterm results after the arterial switch operation for transposition of the great arteries with intact ventricular septum: Clinical, hemodynamic, echocardiographic and electrophysiologic data. Circulation 77:1333–1344

35. Yacoub MH, Radley-Smith R (1978) Anatomy of the coronary arteries in transposition of the great arteries and methods for their transfer in anatomical correction. Thorax 33:418–424

36. Yamaguchi M, Hosokawa Y, Imai Y, Kurosawa H, Yasui H, Yagihara T, Okamoto F, Wakaki N (1990) Early and midterm results of the arterial switch operation for transposition of the great arteries in Japan. J Thorac Cardiovasc Surg 100:261–269

Author's address:
Dr. U. Sauer
Klinik für Herz- und
Kreislauferkrankungen
im Kindesalter
Deutsches Herzzentrum München
Lothstraße 11
8000 München 2

Mustard operation for transposition:
Historical aspects and results

G. A. Trusler
Cardiovascular Surgery, The Hospital for Sick Children, Toronto,
and Department of Surgery, University of Toronto, Toronto, Canada

Historical aspects

Bill Mustard was born, raised and educated in Toronto. He was a fascinating individual: brilliant, proud, ambitious, articulate and extroverted, the life of the party (Fig. 1). We see him as a young surgeon in 1953, playing Santa Claus to the nurses and residents, and at his retirement party in 1976, 23 years later, playing the drums. The fact that he did not know how to play was not important.

After Bill Mustard returned from World War II, he spent a year in the United States completing his training in orthopedic surgery. He joined the staff of the Hospital for Sick Children in 1947 to do both orthopedic and general pediatric surgery. He was an immensely skilled, quick, deft, surgeon, and soon had a busy practice in both areas. At the same time, he was asked to take on the new speciality of cardiovascular surgery which consisted of ductuses, coarctations, and Blalocks. He spent a month in Baltimore observing Blalock and then returned to add this challenge to

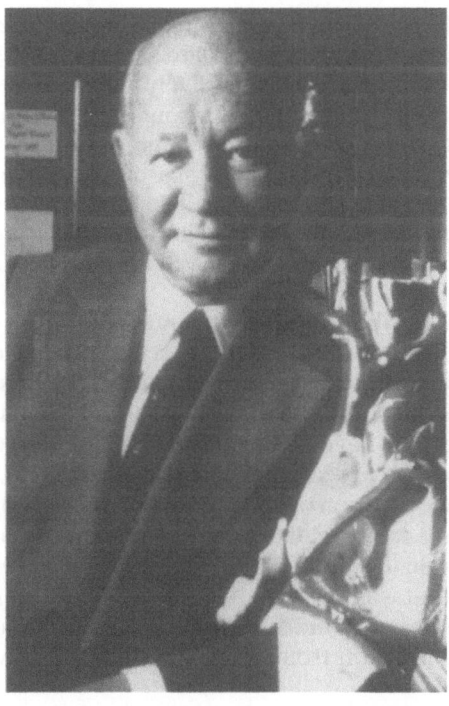

Fig. 1. William Thornton Mustard (1914–1988)

113

his busy life. In 1951 the old hospital, built in 1892, was no longer adequate and they moved to the present building, which has since had two wings added.

At this time, in the laboratory, Mustard was attempting to develop a heart-lung pump and, early on, the challenge of transposition of the great arteries (TGA) appealed to him. In 1952, he operated on seven infants with TGA using a local Campbell Cowan pump with monkey lungs as oxygenators. This experience was published in 1954, and in that paper Mustard described a technique for arterial repair in which only the left coronary artery was transposed [4]. There were no survivors. In that same paper, he described a possible method of partial venous repair wherein the right pulmonary veins were cut from the left atrium and anastomosed to the right atrium and the inferior vena cava was cut from the right atrium and anastomosed to the left atrium. This was not unlike the operation that Baffes described in 1956 [2]. The main difference with Baffes' operation was the use of a graft from the inferior vena cava to the side of the left atrium. I do not believe that Mustard ever tried his operation, but he did try the Baffes procedure without success. In 1959, Senning published his brilliant technique for atrial repair of transposition, but its complexity put it ahead of its time [6]. Bill Mustard did not like complicated, detailed things, but preferred the simple and straight forward. While he admired the Senning operation he did not like its complexity and he was unsuccessful in his few attempts.

Meanwhile, Mustard continued to ponder the problem. His resident at the time, Whit Firor, felt that the inspiration derived from several cases of inadvertent diversion of the vena caval return in the repair of atrial septal defect was the final stimulus to the concept of the Mustard operation. This may indeed be so, although Mustard must also have been aware of the work of Albert [1] and Merendino [3], who described similar procedures.

In May 1963, 28 years ago this month, Mustard did his first Mustard procedure. It was published and presented the following year with immediate acceptance [5]. In the early repairs, the atrial septal defect was enlarged aggressively and quite frequently all of the atrial septum was deliberately removed, cutting outside the heart in order to create a large atrial septal defect. No doubt this accounted for a relatively high initial incidence of postoperative arrhythmias. The pericardial baffle was sutured around the pulmonary veins and then around the cavae. The flow from the cavae was directed to the mitral valve and from the pulmonary veins to the tricuspid valve. The first patient was an infant of 23 months with a small VSD as well as the TGA.

At this point, we must recognize the contribution of the talented Cardiology Department, originally founded and led by John Keith, who gave Bill Mustard great support in his pioneering work. On John Keith's retirement in the mid-1970s, his successor was Dick Rowe, who provided inspired leadership until his retirement and premature death. For the past 5 years, we have been extremely fortunate to have the brilliant and vigorous direction of Bob Freedom, whom you all know.

There were a few changes in the Mustard operation over the years. As the age for surgery was reduced, most cases were done with circulatory arrest. The shape of the baffle gradually changed from a rectangle to something like a dumbbell shape. We reduced the amount of atrial septum that was excised and, in particular, left a ridge of septum medially in an attempt to preserve the artery to the SA node and possibly some preferential channel for conduction from the SA node to the AV node.

Table 1. Repair of complete transposition Hospital for Sick Children 1963–1990

Mustard Procedure	521 children
Rastelli Operation	51 children
Arterial Repair	159 children
Total	731 children

Results

Our total experience to the end of 1990 with repair of transposition of the great arteries other than intraventricular repairs is shown in Table 1. There were a total of 521 Mustard operations. The table depicts the results according to the type of transposition: simple, with VSD, with VSD and PS, and with intact septum and PS, and divides each type into two chronological groups, one before 1974 and the other from 1974 on (Fig. 2). In all types of transposition there was an improvement in results over the years. This is most apparent in the group with simple transposition where there has not been an early death in the last 176 cases. The improvement was least noticeable for the patients with TGA and ventricular septal defects. In the early years, these patients had a high mortality because many of them developed pulmonary vascular disease early, before treatment. There was some improvement with early pulmonary artery banding and a later slight improvement with earlier primary repair, avoiding banding. However, there was still substantial early and late mortality.

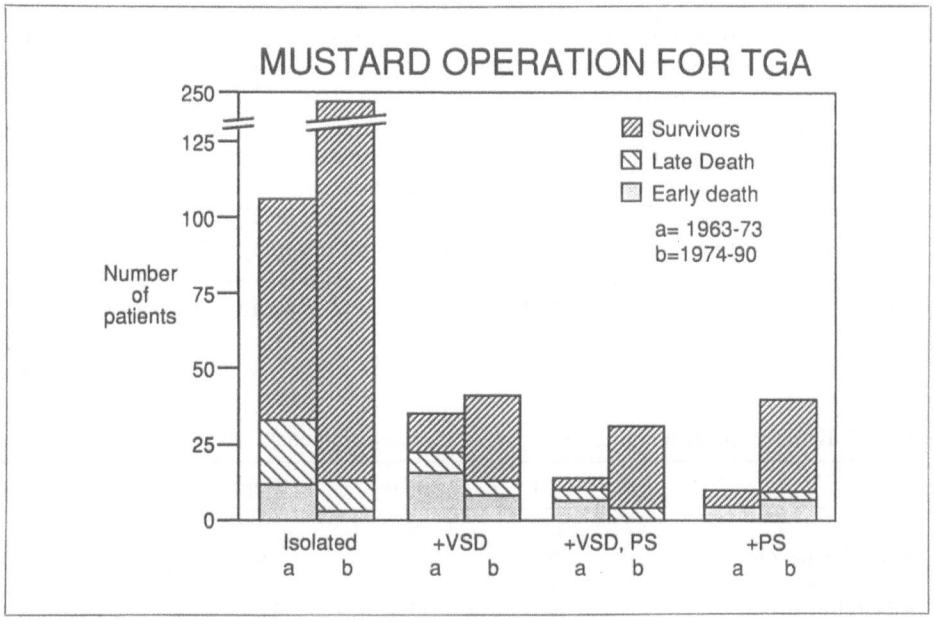

Fig. 2. Graph indicating results for the four anatomic types of transposition over two time periods, 1963–1973 and 1974–1990

115

Furthermore, in surviving patients, the incidence of arrhythmias and right-ventricular dysfunction was higher than in the other groups and, for this reason, in 1978, we started a program of arterial switch repair for patients with transposition and ventricular septal defect.

There was a high mortality in children with the complex, transposition, VSD and pulmonary stenosis. About 1970, these patients were separated into two streams. The main stream was a palliative shunt and later Rastelli repair. The other stream was a very special one for those few infants who had relatively small VSDs and a form of pulmonary stenosis (PS) which could be relieved directly. With appropriate selection, results improved substantially.

Transposition with PS and intact septum is a special small group of patients. The PS may be difficult to relieve and a LV-PA conduit may be required. Results here have also improved over the years.

Complications

The most specific complications of the Mustard operation are the baffle complications, chiefly leaks or venous obstruction (Table 2). With less excision of the atrial septum, the incidence of superior vena caval stenosis remained relatively frequent but inferior caval and pulmonary venous obstructions have decreased. Most obstructions other than pulmonary are relatively mild and do not need surgery, but pulmonary venous obstruction was often fatal and a significant cause of late death. The incidence of surgery for baffle complications was only 25 patients out of 472 survivors, just over 5%.

The largest group, patients with simple or isolated transposition, is also now the most contentious group. In a review of all patients with simple TGA up to the end of 1985, they were divided into two groups, those operated on before 1974 and those from 1974 on [7]. Both early and late deaths were significantly less in the later group. The most dramatic change was a reduction in early mortality to less than 1% and actuarial survival was improved with 94% survival at 10 years. Dysrhythmias have been a problem. Our review of each patient's last electrocardiogram, where available, indicated that over 70% of the second group of patients were in sinus rhythm. Holter ambulatory recording however, showed that while sinus rhythm was present in most, 52% had predominantly junctional rhythms.

Right-ventricular function was also a concern. Almost one-third showed minor diminution in function by angiocardiography or echocardiography, but only 11%

Table 2. Baffle complications (472 survivors − 205 catheterizations)

	Total	Major	Repaired	Died
Shunts	48	8	7	1
SVC Obstruction	37	12	5	
IVC Obstruction	6	2	2	1
PV Obstruction	13	13	11	8
Total	104	35	25	10

appeared to have moderate to severe reduction in right-ventricular function. This was less in the later group of patients, but perhaps that is time-related. Similarly, tricuspid incompetence, usually of mild degree, was noted in 10% of patients studied, some of these in conjunction with right-ventricular dysfunction.

Perhaps the most significant and important facts relate to symptomatology. Those patients operated on after 1973 seem to be doing better than those operated on previously. None of the patients were in NYHA Class III or IV. Most were in Class I with 24% in Class II. Only 21% of patients were on cardiac medication and this was almost entirely for dysrhythmia control. While these results are really not bad, the long-range concern about the right ventricle, and the frequent problems with dysrhythmia have led to a search for some way of achieving a better late functional result, namely the arterial switch operation.

Comments

What are the present indications for the Mustard procedure? Over the past 2 years the presence of pulmonary stenosis was the largest single indication in our hospital, although operating in the newborn period seems to precede or avoid some cases of pulmonary stenosis. We believe that a few rare coronary artery anatomy problems are indications for a Mustard repair. We also believe that age over 4 weeks is an indication until the final results of preliminary pulmonary artery banding are known. Not infrequently, multiple indications exist, but the number of Mustard repairs we do now is very low in comparison with arterial repairs.

Thus, the era of the Mustard operation has largely passed in the short space af about 25 years. You might be interested in knowing of Bill Mustard's first patient. On her 16th birthday she was seen sharing a toast with her surgeon. She now has two children and has had several husbands. She will be 30 years old in June. When examined recently, although her heart size was normal, she was in atrial flutter and she has just had a pacemaker implanted.

Perhaps the message is that all things change and usually for the better. If you come to Toronto 2 years from now you will see another change, a new Hospital for Sick Children, complete with atrium and many other architectural wonders. We hope you will find the occasion to visit us.

References

1. Albert HM (1954) Surgical correction of transposition of the vessels. Surgical Forum 5:74
2. Baffes TG (1956) A new method for surgical correction of transposition of the aorta and pulmonary artery. Surgery, Gynecology and Obstretrics 102:227–233
3. Merendino KA, Jesseph JE, Herron PW et al. (1957) Interatrial venous transposition: A one-stage intracardiac operation for the conversion of complete transposition of the aorta and pulmonary artery. Surgery 42:898
4. Mustard WT, Chute AL, Keith JD, Sirek A, Rowe RD, Vlad P (1954) A surgical approach to transposition of the great vessels with extracorporeal circuit. Surgery 36:39–51
5. Mustard WT (1964) Successful two-stage correction of transposition of the great vessels. Surgery 55:469
6. Senning A (1959) Surgical correction of transposition of the great vessels. Surgery 45:966–980

7. Trusler GA, Williams WG, Duncan KF, Hesslein PS, Benson LN, Freedom RM, Izukawa T, Olley PM (1987) Results with the mustard operation in simple transposition of the great arteries 1963–1985. Ann Surg 206:251–260

Author's address:
George A. Trusler, M.D.
Cardiovascular Surgery
The Hospital for Sick Children
Department of Surgery
University of Toronto
Toronto, Canada

118

Long-term results after atrial repair for transposition of the great arteries

L. K. von Segesser, M. Fry, A. Senning, M. I. Turina
Clinic for Cardiovascular Surgery, University Hospital, Zürich, Switzerland

Introduction

Various procedures have been suggested for correction of transposition of the great arteries, including the techniques developed by Senning [13], Shumacker [14], and Mustard [8] that approach the inlet of the heart, and those proposed by Rastelli [12], Jatene [4] and Damus et al. [1] dealing with the outlet of the heart. Over the years it has become clear that avoiding prosthetic material is of prime importance in order to obtain good long-term results after correction of the growing heart. There are now surgical techniques for repair of transposition of the great arteries that can be performed without use of prosthetic material [17] (despite atrial septostomy [11]) on the atrial level (modified Senning operation [3, 15, 16], as well as on the arterial level (Jatene's procedure in combination with the Lecompte maneuver [2, 6]. However, it is still unknown whether atrial or arterial repair of transposition of the great arteries will finally be superior in the long run. The present study was performed to analyze our long-term results in patients with atrial repair of transposition of the great arteries followed for up to 24 years.

Patients and methods

Long-term results of 254 patients (175 males (69%); 79 females (31%)) surviving 30 days after atrial repair of transposition of the great arteries after 1964 were analyzed. All patients underwent atrial repair as described by Senning [13] and its modifications as previously reported [15, 16]. While mean age at surgery was 6.6 years at the beginning, it decreased progressively to 0.7 years at the end of the 24-year observation period. The analyzed series included 159 (63%) patients with simple transposition of the great arteries and 95 (37%) patients with complex transposition including ventricular septal defects (VSD: 29/95: 31%) and obstruction of the left-ventricular outflow tract (41/95: 43%) or both (25/95: 26%). Long-term survival, cause of death, freedom from pacemaker (PM), and freedom from reoperation were analyzed.

Late mortality was studied in relation to cardiac and non-cardiac death and the former was broken down into failure of the systemic ventricle and sudden death (probably due to arrhythmia). The mean follow-up period was 10.1 years (maximum 24 years). Follow-up comprised 2566 patient years and was, at the time of the study, 95.3% complete. The methods described by Cutler and Ederer were used for actuarial analyses. The results are given with 95% confidence limits.

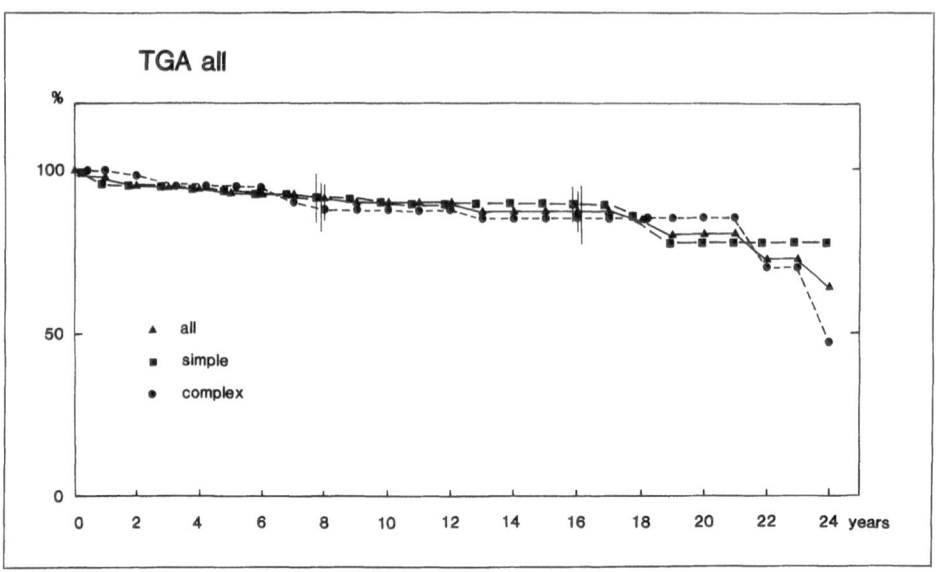

Fig. 1. Actuarial survival curves after repair of transposition of the great arteries (all: n = 254; simple: n = 159; complex: n = 95). Vertical bars indicate 95% confidence limits. At 16 years of follow-up the analyzed groups include 81 patients for all, 58 patients for simple, and 23 patients for complex transpositions.

Results

Overall survival for the complete series was 99.6% after 1 year, 95.4% after 4 years, 91.5% after 8 years, 88.1% after 16 years, and 64.0% after 24 years, as shown in Fig. 1. For the subcategory simple versus complex transposition (Fig. 1) the survival rate was 99.4 vs 100.0% for 1 year, 93.8% vs 88.3% for 8 years, 89.6% vs 85.8% for 16 years, 85.1% vs 85.8% for 18 years, and 77.7% vs 46.8% at 24 years.

Freedom from pacemaker implantation (PM) after atrial correction of transposition of the great arteries is depicted in Fig. 2 and applied to 98.4% after 1 year, 96.6% after 4 years, 95.1% after 8 years, 90.5% after 16 years, and 87.1% after 24 years.

Freedom from reoperation (excluding pacemakers) after atrial correction of transposition of the great arteries is shown in Fig. 3. After 1 year, 99.6% of the patients had not been reoperated and the respective figures are 94.9% after 4 years, 93.5% after 8 years, 87.1% after 16 years, and 87.1% after 24 years.

Actuarial survival in patients not requiring reoperations is given in Fig. 4. In this group, the survival rate was 99.6% after 1 year, 95.9% after 4 years, 92.5% after 8 years, 90.3% after 16 years, and 65.0% after 24 years.

The analysis of 37 late deaths showed that there were 28/37 cardiac deaths (68%) including 14/37 systemic ventricle failures (38%) and 9/37 sudden deaths (24%). Systemic ventricle failure and sudden death accounted for 11 deaths in 159 patients with simple transposition (7%) and 12 deaths in 95 patients with complex transposition of the great arteries (13%). Other causes of death included infection (5/37), accident (2/37), and unknown (2/37).

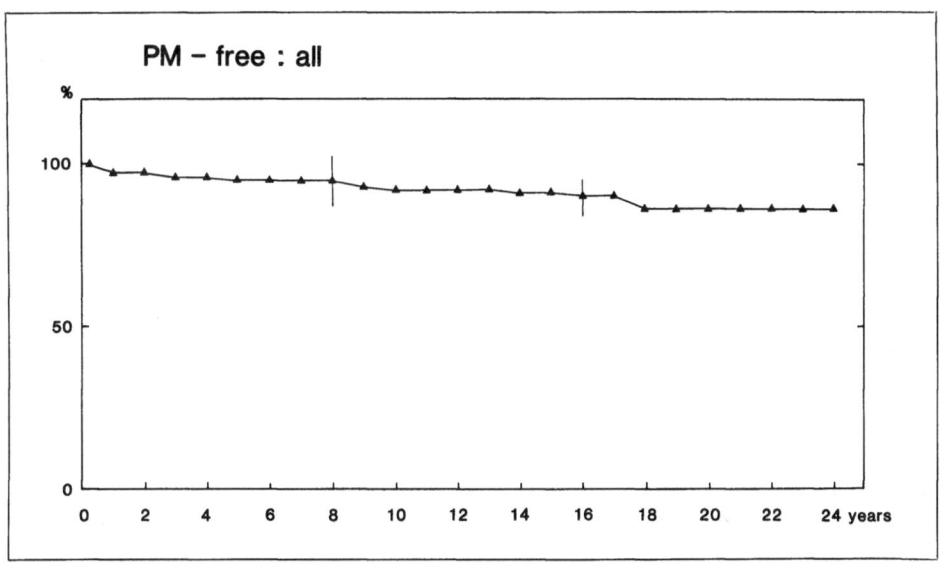

Fig. 2. Actuarial freedom from pacemarker (PM) in patients who underwent atrial repair of transposition of the great arteries. Vertical bars indicate 95% confidence limits. At 16-year follow-up there remain 78 patients to be analyzed.

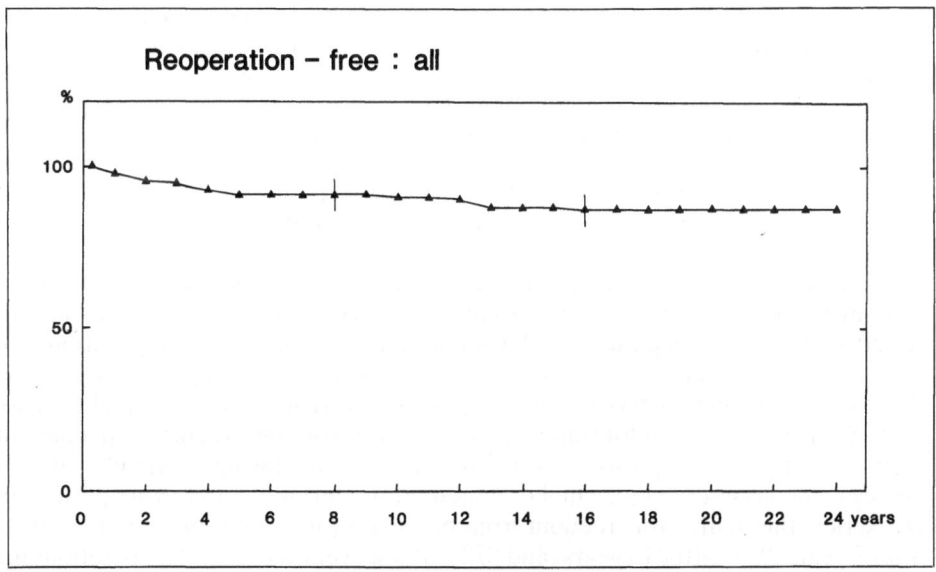

Fig. 3. Actuarial freedom from reoperation after atrial repair of transposition of the great arteries. Vertical bars indicate 95% confidence limits. At 16-year follow-up, there remain 72 patients to be analyzed.

121

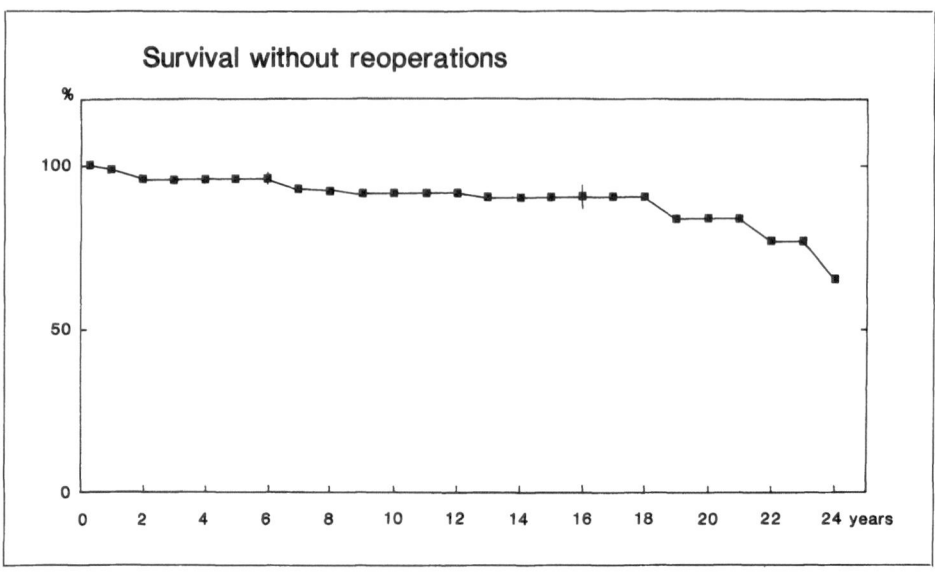

Fig. 4. Actuarial survival curve after atrial repair of transposition of the great arteries, excluding patients requiring reoperations. Vertical bars indicate 95% confidence limits. After 16 years there remain 74 patients to be followed up.

Discussion

Long-term follow-up of our patients operated since 1964 showed remarkable survival rates of over 91% at 8 years and 88% at 16 years. In simple transposition the results are even better and account for over 93% after 8 years, and 89% after 16 years. Survival after 24 years of follow-up is 77.7% for simple versus 46.8% for complex transpositions (Fig. 1). It is difficult to assess whether the inferior results for complex transpositions are due to the type of correction or due to the associated lesions, particularly since, in the early years, a large number of patients with transposition of the great arteries never went to surgery and the surgical population was highly selective.

Obviously, systemic ventricular failure and sudden death are the main complications in the long-term evolution of the patients undergoing atrial correction of transposed great vessels. In patients with simple transposition, these complications are about half as frequent (7%) as compared to patients with complex transposition (13%), resulting in a linearized rate of systemic ventricle failure and sudden death of 0.28% per patient year for simple transposition as compared to 0.54% per patient year for complex transpositions. One indicator for increasing ventricular insufficiency is the necessity of pacemaker implantation during the follow-up period. In our series, the figures for freedom from pacemaker implantation were over 95% after 8 years, 90% after 16 years, and 87% after 24 years (Fig. 2). Reoperations for tricuspid regurgitation (i.e., the atrioventricular valve on the systemic side) are another indicator for ongoing systemic ventricular failure. For our series, those for freedom from reoperation (excluding pacemakers) were over 93% after 8 years,

122

87% after 16 years, and 87% after 24 years (Fig. 3). As a result, it is not surprising that the survival rate for patients without reoperation is somewhat better than that for the complete series. At this time, the review of the literature shows an expected survival rate for simple transposition of 84.2% at 18 years [7] as compared to 85.1% at 18 years and 77.7% at 24 years in this series. The expected survival of 96.1% after 2 years in this series compares favorably with the 96% survival after arterial switch reported by the Congenital Heart Surgeons Society [9] (perioperative mortality was excluded for both series).

For transposition of the great arteries with VSD the Congenital Heart Surgeons Society [9] reports for the arterial-switch operation (n = 29) a 2-year survival rate of 100% which matches exactly the 100% survival rate at 2 years of this series (Fig. 1). Quaegebeur [10] reported for his series of arterial-switch operations a survival rate of 81% at 11 months and no mortality thereafter for patients traced up to 8 years. A 90% survival rate at 2 years is finally reported for the Damus-Kaye-Stansel operation [1] which may be useful in some cases with prepared left ventricle.

Hence, at this time, atrial repair of transposition of the great arteries appears to be a valid approach for simple transpositions of the great arteries. There is still no proof of superior long-term results for the arterial or so-called anatomical correction of transposition because of the unknown fate of the subpulmonary valve in aortic position and transposed coronary artery ostia and proximal coronary arteries. It has to be further considered that in recent years, surgical results have been improved for all, i.e., the arterial as well as the atrial corrections of transposed great arteries.

References

1. Ceithaml EL, Puga FJ, Danielson GK, McGoon DC, Ritter DG (1984) Results of the Damus-Stansel-Kaye procedure for transposition of the great arteries and for double outlet right ventricle with subpulmonary ventricular septal defect. Ann Thorac Surg 38:433–437
2. Dunn JM (1991) Jatene's arterial repair for transposition of the great vessels. Ann Thorac Surg 51:511–514
3. Ingram MT, von Segesser LK, Ott DA, Huhta JC, Murphy Jr DJ (1988) Senning repair for transposition of the great arteries without patch augmentation of the septum. J Thorac Cardiovasc Surg 96:485–487
4. Jatene AD, Fontes VF, Paulista PP (1976) Anatomic correction of transposition of the great vessels. J Thorac Cardiovasc Surg 72:364–370
5. Kron IL, Rheuban KS, Joob AW, Jedeiken R, Mentzer RM, Carpenter MA, Nolan SP (1985) Baffle obstruction following the Mustard operation: cause and treatment. Ann Thorac Surg 39:112–115
6. Lecompte Y, Zannini L, Hazan E et al. (1981) Anatomic correction of transposition of the great arteries: New technique without use of a prosthetic conduit. J Thorac Cardiovasc Surg 82:629–631
7. Merlo M, De Tommasi SM, Brunelli F, Abbruzzese PA, Crupi G, Ghidoni I, Casari A, Piti A, Mamprin F, Parenzan L (1991) Long term results after atrial correction of complete transposition of the great arteries. Ann Thorac Surg 51:227–231
8. Mustard WT (1964) Successful two-stage correction of transposition of the great vessels. Surgery 55:469–472
9. Norwood WI, Dobell AR, Freed MD, Kirklin JW, Blackstone EH and the Congenital Heart Surgeons Society (1988) Intermediate results of the arterial switch repair. J Thorac Cardiovasc Surg 96:854–863
10. Quaegebeur JM, Rohmer J, Ottenkamp J et al. (1986) The arterial switch operation: An eight year experience. J Thorac Cardiovasc Surg 92:361–384

11. Rashkind WJ, Miller WW (1968) Transposition of the great arteries: Results of palliation by balloon atrioseptostomy in 31 patients. Circulation 38:453
12. Rastelli GC, Wallace RB, Ongley PA (1969) Complete repair of transposition of the great arteries with pulmonary stenosis: A review and report of a case corrected by using a new surgical technique. Circulation 39:83
13. Senning A (1959) Surgical correction of transposition of the great vessels. Surgery 45:966–980
14. Shumacker HB (1961) A new operation for transposition of the great vessels. Surgery 50:773–777
15. Siebenmann R, von Segesser LK, Schneider K, Schneider J, Senning A, Turina M (1989) Late failure of systemic ventricle after atrial correction for transposition of great arteries. Eur J Cardiothorac Surg 3:119–124
16. Turina M, Siebenmann R, Nussbaumer P, Senning A (1988) Long-term outlook after atrial correction of transposition of great arteries. J Thorac Cardiovasc Surg 95:828–835
17. von Segesser LK, Jornod N, Faidutti B, Turina M (1989) Indications for pericardial xenograft in repair of congenital heart disease. J Cardiac Surgery 4:149–155

Author's address:
Ludwig K. von Segesser, MD
Clinic for Cardiovascular Surgery
University Hospital
CH-8091 Zürich, Switzerland

The "rapid two-stage" arterial switch operation

A. R. Castaneda

Cardiac Surgery Dept., The Children's Hospital, Boston, Massachusetts, USA

Introduction

In transposition of the great arteries and intact ventricular septum (TGA/IVS), left-ventricular (LV) muscle mass is normal at birth. However, the rapidly decreasing pulmonary vascular resistance results in a drop of peak LV pressure and, consequently, decreased development of LV muscle mass. Approximately by 1 month of age, most patients with TGA/IVS have a peak LV/RV pressure ratio equal to or less than 0.6. Therefore, in patients with TGA/IVS, we prefer to perform the arterial switch operation (ASO) ideally during the first few weeks of life when the LV is still prepared to support the systemic circulation [1]. Since this is not always possible, we base our decision to do an ASO on arbitrary criteria. Before 2 weeks of age, all patients with TGA/IVS have repair regardless of preoperative hemodynamics. After 2 weeks of age, an LV/RV pressure ratio of 0.6 is accepted as the lower limit for an ASO. Helpful, but not yet absolutely defined are two-dimensional echocardiographic indices of a left ventricle suitable for ASO, including ventricular septal position, degree of LV wall-thickness, LV volume, and LV muscle mass. If the LV/RV ratio is less than 0.6, the LV must be "prepared" to assume the function of a systemic ventricle.

In 1989, we reported [2] our first results of surgical treatment of an initial group of 11 patients with TGA/IVS (or a restrictive VSD) who had undergone a "rapid two-stage arterial switch procedure" which included a short period (median 7 days) between banding of the main pulmonary artery and the ASO. The most common indication for the procedure was 1) referral to our center after the neonatal period, 2) multiorgan failure in the neonatal period which contraindicated corrective surgery, 3) prematurity, and 4) late development of right-ventricular dysfunction which contraindicated correction at the atrial level originally planned at the referral center. This report is an update on our experience with the rapid two-stage arterial switch procedure.

Methods

The initial operation consists of interposition of a modified 4-mm Blalock-Taussig shunt between the right subclavian artery and the right pulmonary artery, either through a right thoracotomy or median sternotomy, and banding of the pulmonary trunk until LV pressure rises to approximately 75% of the systemic pressure. The child is then returned to the intensive care unit for approximately 1 week before the shunt and the band are taken down and the ASO is accomplished. Serial echocardiograms during this period demonstrate a dramatic increase in LV muscle mass

125

(mean increase 85%) usually within 3 to 5 days. The LV ejection fraction tends to be depressed during the first 3 days, during which time the patients often required inotropic support. Generally, by day 7, the LV ejection fraction has returned to normal. These clinical findings are consistent with experimental data where extremely rapid induction of c-fos and c-myc proto-oncogenes has been demonstrated within 1 h after imposition of an acute ventricular pressure load [3]. Likewise, the genes responsible for the adaptive response of the isozymes of rat myocardial myosin, actin, and tropomyosin are maximally induced within 48 h under similar circumstances [4].

The second stage, that is the ASO, requires no modification relative to the procedure performed as a primary operation other than division of the Blalock shunt and removal of the band. There is no need to place, for example, a conduit from the right ventricle to the pulmonary trunk as has been described by others who have undertaken the two-stage switch with a longer period of 6 to 12 months between palliation and correction [5].

As of July, 1991, 31 patients have undergone the "rapid two-stage arterial switch operation" at Children' Hospital, Boston. Median age at the time of the ASO was 4 months with a range of 4 weeks to 21 months. There was one death during the interval between palliation and correction. This child was born prematurely, weighing 1600 grams and had previously undergone repair of an aortic coarctation. The child was known to have significant pulmonary pathology and at post-mortem was found to have stenosis of both left and right upper lobe pulmonary veins. There also was one early death after the ASO in a child who had aortic thrombi preoperatively. Following a technically satisfactory ASO, this child suffered a sudden cardiac arrest, 36 h after the repair. An acute thrombus was found within the aortic arch at post-mortem examination.

Mean follow-up of the survivors is 29 months (range 1 to 47 months). In all 13 patients who have undergone postoperative catheterization, LV function, both systolic and diastolic, was normal. Electrophysiologic studies in 9 patients showed normal sinus and A-V node function.

Conclusion

We are encouraged by our experience so far with the "rapid two-stage arterial switch procedure". Preliminary pulmonary artery banding is effective in increasing left-ventricular afterload, and the modified Blalock-Taussig shunt provides an adequate pulmonary blood flow. Both stages can be performed during one hospitalization. In addition to the advantages of less distortion of the pulmonary trunk and neo-aortic valve by the short-term pulmonary artery band, and also the greater ease at reoperation because of fewer adhesions, there are also psychosocial, logistic, and financial benefits from this approach.

References

1. Castaneda AR, Norwood WI, Jonas RA, Colon SD, Sanders SP, Lang P (1984) Transposition of the great arteries and intact ventricular septum: anatomical repair in the neonate. Ann Thorac Surg 38:438–443

2. Jonas RA, Giglia TM, Sanders SP, Wernovsky G, Nadal-Ginard B, Mayer JE, Castaneda AR (1989) Rapid, two-stage arterial switch for transposition of the great arteries and intact ventricular septum beyond the neonatal period. Circulation 80 (Suppl I):I 203−208
3. Izumo S, Nadal-Ginard B, Mahdavi V (1988) Protooncogene induction and reprogramming of cardiac gene expression produced by pressure overload. Proc Natl Acad Sci USA 85:339−343
4. Izumo S, Lompre AM, Matsuoka R, Koren G, Schwarta K, Nadan-Ginard B, Mahdavi V (1987) Myosin heavy chain messenger RNA and protein isoform transitions during cardiac hypertrophy. J Clin Invest 79:970−977
5. Yacoub MH, Bernhard A, Lange P, Radley-Smith R, Keck E, Stephan E, Heintzen P (1980) Clinical and hemodynamic results of the two-stage anatomic correction of simple transposition of the great arteries. Circulation 62 (Suppl I):I 190−196

Author's address:
Aldo R. Castaneda, M.D.
Cardiac Surgery Department
The Children's Hospital
300 Longwood Avenue
Boston, MA 02115

Anatomic repair for complex transposition

Y. Lecompte[1], F. Bourlon[1], K. Hisatomi[2], D. Di Carlo[3]
[1]Centre Cardio-Thoracique de Monaco, Monaco Cedex
[2]Kurume University School of Medicine, Kurume-shi Japan
[3]Ospedale Bambino Gesù, Rome, Italy

Introduction

During the last 15 years, the development of the arterial switch procedure has radically modified the approach to all types of transposition of the great arteries. As soon as the technical difficulties were overcome, this procedure was diffusely applied to the treatment of patients with transposition associated with ventricular septal defect (VSD) for two orders of reason: first, in these patients, the left ventricle was adapted to its systemic function; second, the results of the atrial switch were unsatisfactory in this subset. Subsequently, the true revolution was the large-scale application of the arterial switch operation to patients with simple transposition when it became understood that the neo-natal period was, because of physiologic reasons, the optimal age for this repair. Even if the long-term fate of this procedure remains unknown, this approach is today commonly endorsed. However, in the domain of transposition of the great arteries, a few complex lesions are left for which the best form of repair is still debated. This review is concerned with three of these forms: transposition with pulmonary stenosis without ventricular septal defect (VSD), transposition with straddling tricuspid valve, and transposition with VSD and pulmonary stenosis.

Transposition of the great arteries with pulmonary stenosis and without VSD

The association of a severe pulmonary stenosis with transposition of the great arteries is very rare in the absence of a VSD. Generally, the subpulmonary obstruction, in transposition with intact ventricular septum, is either dynamic or due to the leftward deviation of the infundibular septum. In these cases, the pulmonary valve is normal. It is accepted that this common type of subpulmonary stenosis does not contraindicate an atrial nor an arterial switch. However, some patients present at repair with fibro-muscular subpulmonary obstruction without VSD. The majority of these children are beyond the neonatal age, and it is conceivable that this association may be the result of spontaneous closure of a VSD present at birth. We treated, in 1979, this anomaly in a 3-month-old baby. The technique of translocation of the entire aortic root described by Bex [1], and subsequently by Nikhaido [5] was used, and was associated with the transection of the hypoplastic pulmonary annulus. The infundibular septum was divided and the aortic root was reimplanted on the widely open left-ventricular outflow tract. Twelve years later, the patient is asymptomatic. At control catheterization, 6 years after repair, normal pressures and function of both ventricles were found. Surgeons should be aware of this technique for repairing this ominous anomaly but, unlike Nikhaido [5], we do not

129

advocate its use in cases associated with VSD, for whom, even when the defect is restrictive, simpler and safer solutions are available.

Transposition of the great arteries with straddling tricuspid valve

Severe degrees of straddling of the tricuspid valve (i.e., insertion of chordae on a left-sided papillary muscle and not simply on the left surface of the interventricular septum) are generally regarded as a contraindication for an arterial switch. We recently performed an anatomic repair on two patients with this anomaly. The first one was 5 months of age. The stradding leaflet was attached by a few short chordae to the crest of the interventricular septum. These were transected. The VSD was subsequently closed by a patch which was anchored, in part to the valvar tissue and in part to the septum: half of the defect was thus closed by the patch, the other half by the leaflet itself. The post-operative course was uncomplicated.

Encouraged by this case, we subsequently operated on a child in whom a pulmonary arterial band had been placed during the neo-natal period and for whom an arterial switch had been considered inadvisable for 10 years. In this case, the left-sided insertions of the tricuspid valve were anteriorly located and caused sub-pulmonary obstruction. The chordae were severed, in order to prevent the occurrence of subaortic stenosis after the arterial switch, and the leaflet was directly sutured to the interventricular septum, thus completely closing the VSD. These two patients enjoy an excellent functional result, free of significant tricuspid regurgitation. The first one, who had had no disturbance of the atrio-ventricular (AV) conduction in the early post-operative period, developed a complete AV block, 3 months after surgery, probably related to the anatomic anomalies of the AV junction. This limited experience suggests that a straddling tricuspid valve is not a contraindication, per se, for an arterial switch procedure. However, most of these valvar anomalies are associated with right-ventricular hypoplasia and this may represent a true contraindication to anatomic repair in these patients.

Transposition of the great arteries associated with VSD and pulmonary stenosis

In 1981, we [4] described a technique called "réparation à l'étage ventriculaire" or REV, the aim of which was to avoid the restrictions inherent to the Rastelli procedure [6]. These are summarized in Fig. 1A. Principles and theoretical advantages of the REV procedure are shown in Fig. 1B.

From November 1980 to March 1991, 92 patients underwent this operation: 56 for "classic" transposition of the great arteries and 36 for other types of ventriculo-arterial connection not amenable to intraventricular repair [2]. Their age at operation is indicated in Fig. 2. About two-thirds of the patients were younger than 5 years at surgery and 40% were younger than two years. Forty-three patients had undergone a previous palliative procedure (Table 1). The three patients with previous pulmonary banding could not be candidate for an arterial switch: one had a sub-pulmonary stenosis of a degree inadequate to protect the pulmonary arterial bed but, nonetheless, incompatible with a safe repair at arterial level; in the two other patients, who presented to our institution late in their natural history, pulmonary valve insufficiency had resulted from banding of the pulmonary artery. The

130

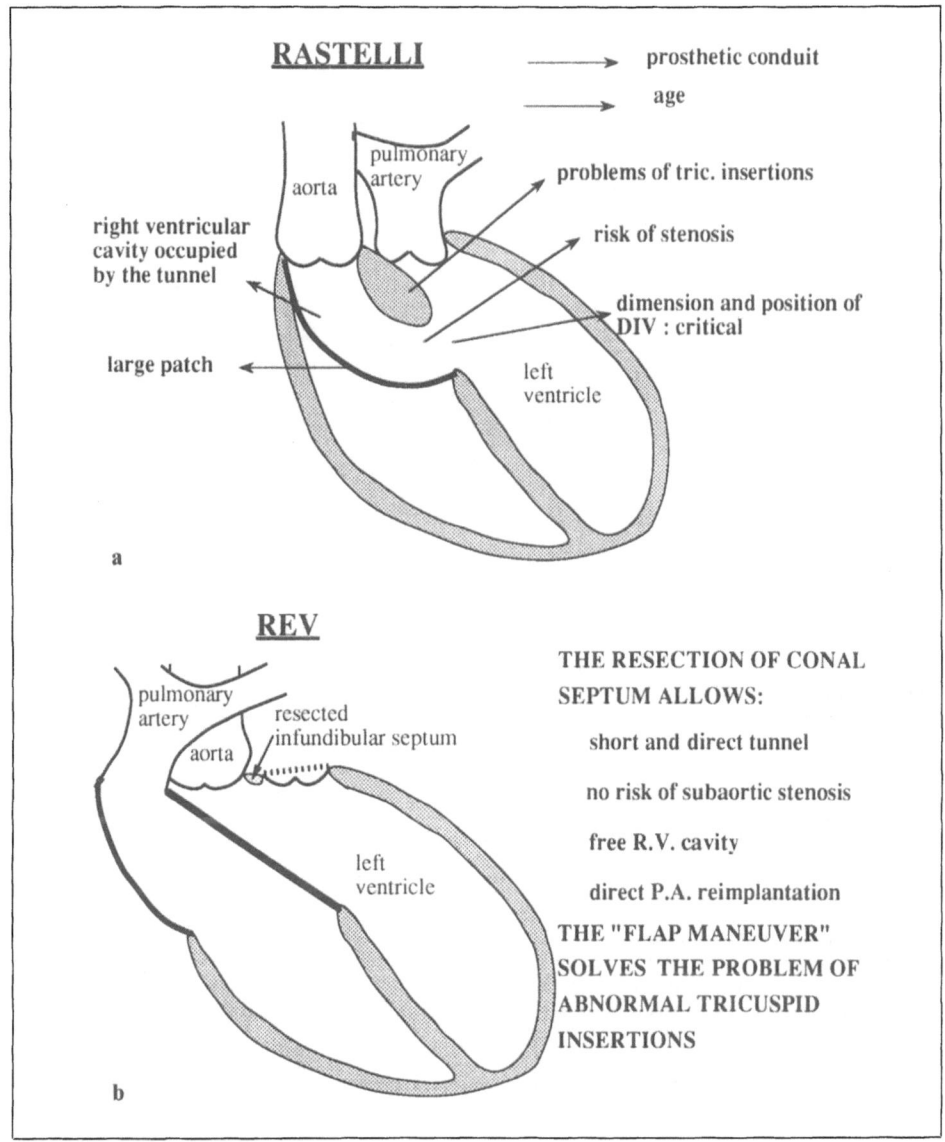

RASTELLI ————→ prosthetic conduit

————→ age

aorta / pulmonary artery

problems of tric. insertions

right ventricular cavity occupied by the tunnel

risk of stenosis

dimension and position of DIV : critical

large patch

left ventricle

a

REV

pulmonary artery

resected infundibular septum

aorta

left ventricle

THE RESECTION OF CONAL SEPTUM ALLOWS:

short and direct tunnel

no risk of subaortic stenosis

free R.V. cavity

direct P.A. reimplantation

THE "FLAP MANEUVER" SOLVES THE PROBLEM OF ABNORMAL TRICUSPID INSERTIONS

b

Fig. 1.

associated anomalies are listed in Table 2. The most common was the insertion of tricuspid chordae on the infundibular septum. In these cases, the septum was not resected, but was mobilized posteriorly, together with the anomalous valvar insertions ("flap maneuver"), as previously described [2]. The prevalence of restrictive VSDs in this series is probably underestimated in the data presented in Table 2, since we included only the cases in whom a supra-systemic left-ventricular pressure was found. In several others, the VSD was smaller than the aortic orifice. One of

131

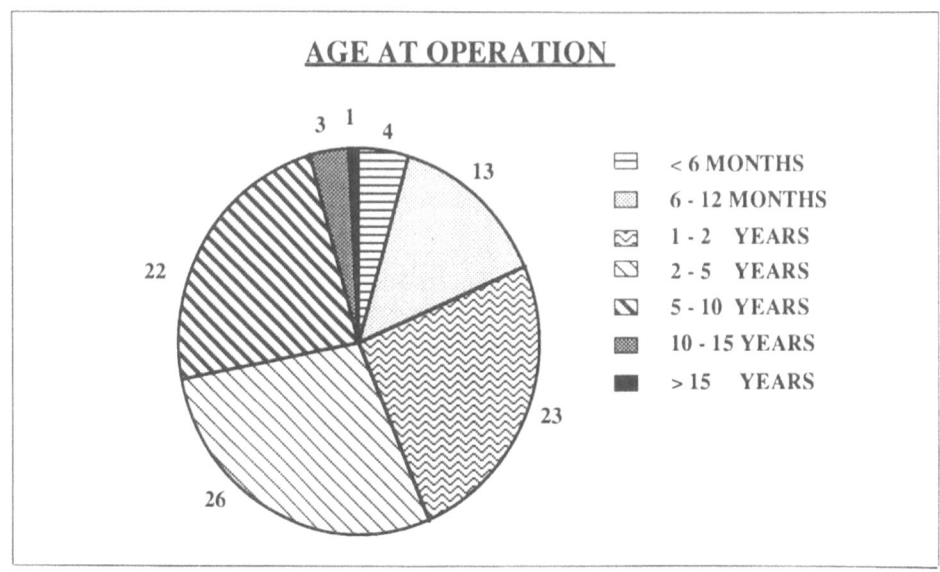

Fig. 2

Table 1. Previous palliation

37 Patients	1 Shunt
3 Patients	2 Shunts
3 Patients	PA banding

Table 2. Associated anomalies

17:	Tricuspid chordae on the infundibular septum
2:	Straddling tricuspid valve
7:	Multiple VSD's
9:	Restrictive VSD

the foremost benefits of the septal resection is that the size of the intracardiac tunnel is not affected by the dimension of the VSD. No patient in our experience was contraindicated because of a small VSD.

The overall mortality in our whole experience was 15% (Table 3). It was higher in patients younger than 1 year at operation. However, age may not be a risk factor per se, since many of these babies had major associated defects. Young age at surgery, which significantly increased the hazard for death early in our experience, no longer represents an incremental risk factor, probably due to better patient-selection: we now decline patients with severe hypoplasia of either the left ventricle or of the pulmonary arterial bed. During the last 10 years, the hospital mortality

Table 3. Hospital deaths

Total 14/92	15%
Under 1 year	29%
Above 1 year	12%
First 3 years experience	25%
Last 7 years	10%

Table 4. Causes of hospital deaths

Left ventricle + pulmonary art. hypoplasia	4
Insufficient septal resection	2
Coronary artery injury	2
Sepsis	2
Residual VSD	1
Hemoptysis	1
"Low output"	2
	14

Table 5. Reoperations

From 8 days to 10 years after repair	
Residual VSD	2
Residual VSD + pulm. stenosis	1
VSD + tricuspid insufficiency	2
VSD + tric. insuf. + pulm. sten.	2
Pulmonary stenosis	1
	8

was 10%. The causes of the hospital deaths are listed in Table 4. In most cases, a wrong indication or technical mistakes were implicated which could be, theoretically, avoided.

Three late deaths have occurred. One was probably due to ventricular arythmia, 1 year after repair, in a child with preoperative marked left-ventricular hypertrophy secondary to a restrictive VSD (systolic left-ventricular pressure at rest >200 mmHg). Residual obstruction had been excluded by catheterization a few weeks before death. Another patient probably succumbed to sudden dysfunction of a permanent pace-maker implanted for postoperative AV block. The last patient died after heart transplantation. This patient had suffered a perioperative myocardial infarction and developed progressive myocardial failure.

Eight patients have required reoperation. The causes of reintervention are listed in Table 5. Three types of complications were observed: residual VSD, tricuspid regurgitation, and pulmonary stenosis. Residual VSD is a well-known drawback of this type of repair and our technique is not an exception. Tricuspid insufficiency, remarkably, did not develop in any patient with abnormal tricuspid insertions. In

133

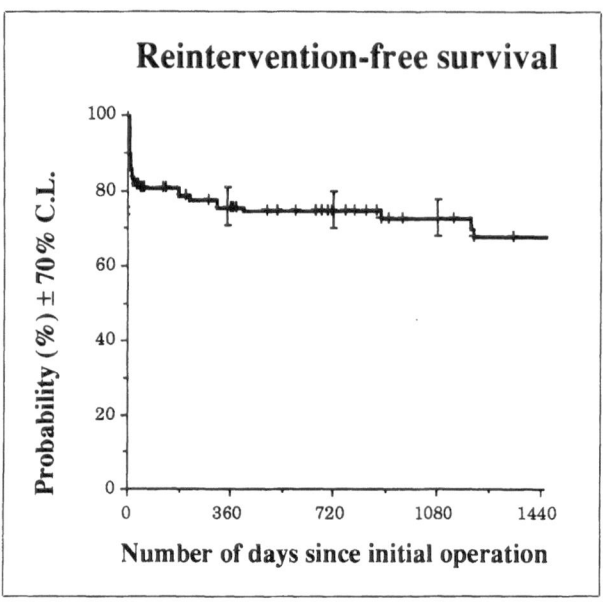

Fig. 3

Table 6. Left ventricular function

	REV	Rastelli	Normal
Normal L. V. stress	15/22	3/11	
Telediast. volume	68	104	60
Ejection fraction	60%	53%	63%

all cases, this complication could be repaired with conservative procedures. Finally, pulmonary stenosis seemed to be related to imperfect reconstruction rather than to lack of growth of the pulmonary tract, since it was usually observed shortly after repair and was independent of age of the patients. The probability of freedom from death and reoperation is represented by the Kaplan Meyer method in Fig. 3.

All patients, including those who underwent reoperation, were in functional class I at the time of this review. During the follow-up period, we have not observed progressive subaortic obstruction in any case. In all patients, size and function of the left ventricle appear normal. We recently investigated more specifically the left-ventricular function in 22 patients, employing the echocardiographic method proposed by Graham et al. [3] for assessing the results of the Rastelli operation. In Table 6, we compare the data obtained from our patients with those reported by the above-mentioned authors and with values from the normal subjects. With reference to the three parameters which were abnormal after the Rastelli procedure, the REV series is more similar to normal controls. The exact explanation of this fact is unknown, but it can be supposed that the smaller size of the intra-ventricular patch, the avoidance of residual subaortic stenosis, and the younger age of our patients play a role determining these differences.

In conclusion, it must be emphasized that, along with simple transposition and transposition with VSD, other complex forms of transposition are amenable to an anatomic repair, which offers the best chance of a good long-term result.

References

1. Bex JP, Lecompte Y, Baillot F, Hazan E (1980) Anatomical correction of transposition of the great arteries. Ann Thorac Surg 29:86–88
2. Borromée L, Lecompte Y, Batisse A, Lemoine G, Vouhé P, Sakata R, Leca F, Zannini L, Neveux JY (1988) Anatomic repair of anomalies of ventriculo-arterial connection associated with ventricular septal defect. II. Clinical results in 50 patients with pulmonary outflow tract obstruction. J Thorac Cardiovasc Surg 95:96–102
3. Graham TP Jr, Franklin RCG, Wise RKH, Gooch V, Deanfield JE (1987) Left ventricle wall stress and contractile function in transposition of the great arteries after the Rastelli operation. J Thorac Cardiovasc Surg 93:775–784
4. Lecompte Y, Neveux JY, Leca F, Zannini L, Tran Viet Tu, Duboys Y, Jarreau MM (1982) Reconstruction of the pulmonary outflow tract without prosthetic conduit. J Thorac Cardiovasc Surg 84:727–733
5. Nikaidoh H (1984) Aortic translocation and biventricular outflow tract reconstruction. A new surgical repair for transposition of the great arteries associated with ventricular septal defect and pulmonary stenosis. J Thorac Cardiovasc Surg 88:365–372
6. Rastelli GC (1969) A new approach to "anatomic" repair of transposition of the great arteries. Mayo Clin Proc 44:1–12
7. Sakata R, Lecompte Y, Batisse A, Borromée L, Durandy Y (1988) Anatomic repair of anomalies of ventriculo-arterial connection associated with ventricular septal defect. I. Criteria of surgical decision. J Thorac Cardiovasc Surg 95:90–95

Author's address:
Y. Lecompte
Centre Cardio-Thoracique de Monaco
11 bis Avenue d'Ostende
MC 98004 Monaco Cedex

Re-operations after surgery for transposition of the great arteries

J. Stark
Cardiothoracic Unit, The Hospital for Sick Children, London, England

Introduction

A tremendous progress has been achieved in the surgical treatment of transposition of the great arteries (TGA), since 1966, when Rashkind and Miller [3] published their work on balloon septostomy. Some old operations were refined and the new operations developed. However, despite all the progress there are still patients who develop early or late problems and who require help. The problems can occur after atrial-type operations such as Mustard or Senning operation, but also after the anatomic-type of repair such as Rastelli or Jatene operation. Some complications can be treated medically, others require surgical treatment. I will briefly describe various surgical complications and the techniques we use to treat them.

Complications after atrial repair for simple transposition

The following problems were described: Systemic venous obstruction, pulmonary venous obstruction, residual or recurrent left-ventricular outflow tract obstruction, right-ventricular failure and baffle leaks. Some of these complications could perhaps be avoided. Meticulous surgical technique, appropriate perfusion and myocardial preservation techniques at the first operation provide the best prevention. However, when these complications do occur treatment is necessary. Systemic venous obstruction after Mustard operation was described from several centres from the early 1970s. It was thought to be related to the surgical technique, possibly also to the material used for the baffle. If more than 50% of the pathway is formed by a patch, subsequent constriction of the patch may cause obstruction. After Senning operation systemic venous obstruction is extremely rare in our experience. The diagnosis of obstruction could be made by echo/Doppler, but the detailed visualisation of the pathways is best done by angiocardiography. Systemic venous obstruction used to be treated surgically, however, some of the ideas of Bill Rashkind prompted the use of balloons in other areas, i.e. not only pulling them across the atrial septum. Figure 1 shows severe IVC obstruction and its relief by balloon dilatation.

If the dilatation is not successful surgical help may be required. We have always approached this and other complications in transposition through the right anterolateral thoracotomy which gives excellent approach compared to redo sternotomy (Fig. 2). From sternotomy injury to the anteriorly placed right ventricle and coronary arteries can occur. In addition, dissection of the SVC and IVC in the presence of high pressure collaterals may be more cumbersome from the sternotomy. From the right-sided approach the aorta, SVC and IVC are easily dis-

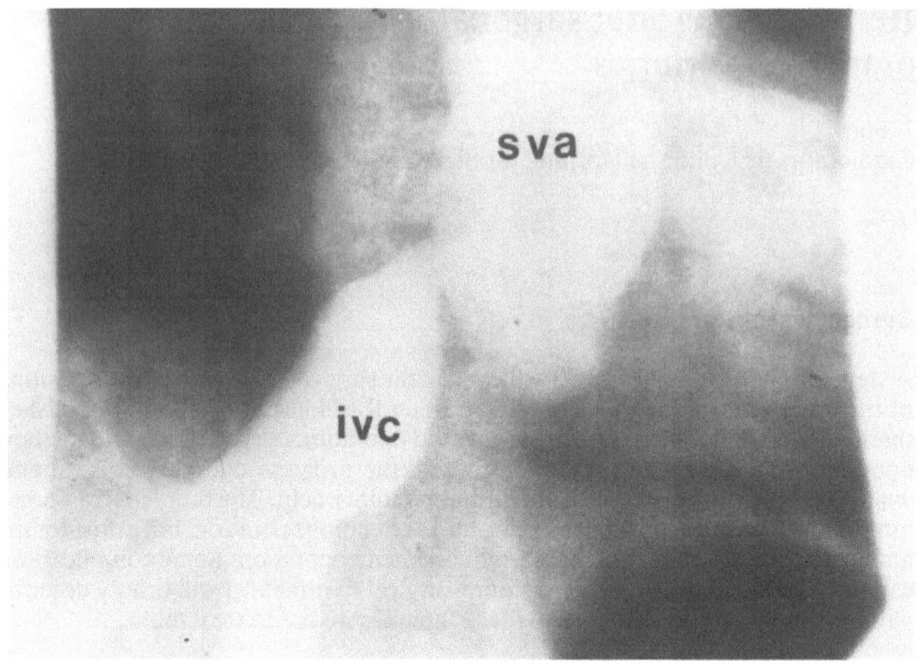

Fig. 1a. IVC angio demonstrates severe obstruction of the IVC pathway. IVC – inferior vena cava; SVC – systemic vena cava.

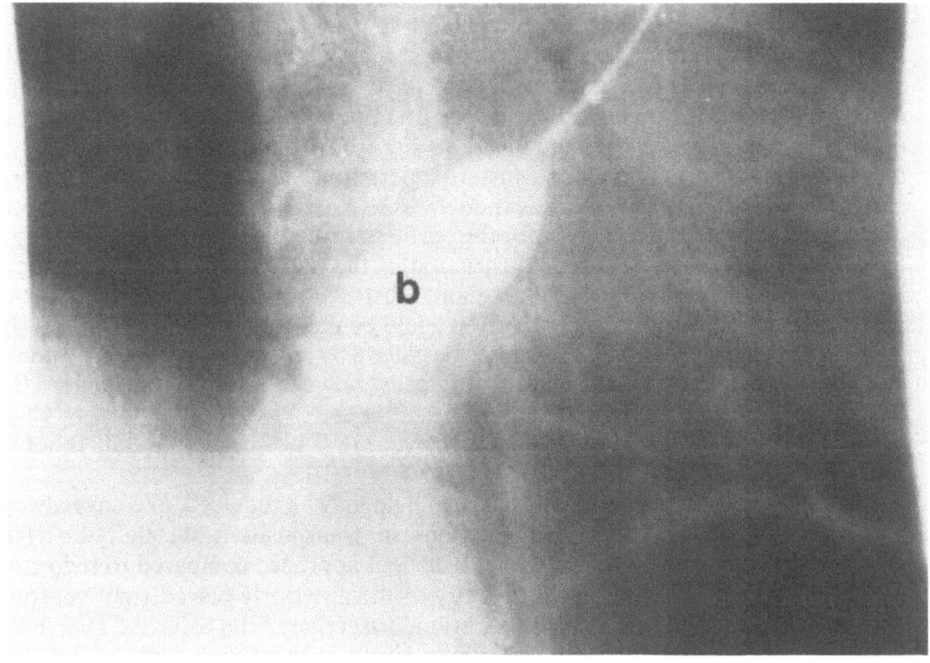

Fig. 1b. Balloon is dilated in the area of obstruction. B – balloon.

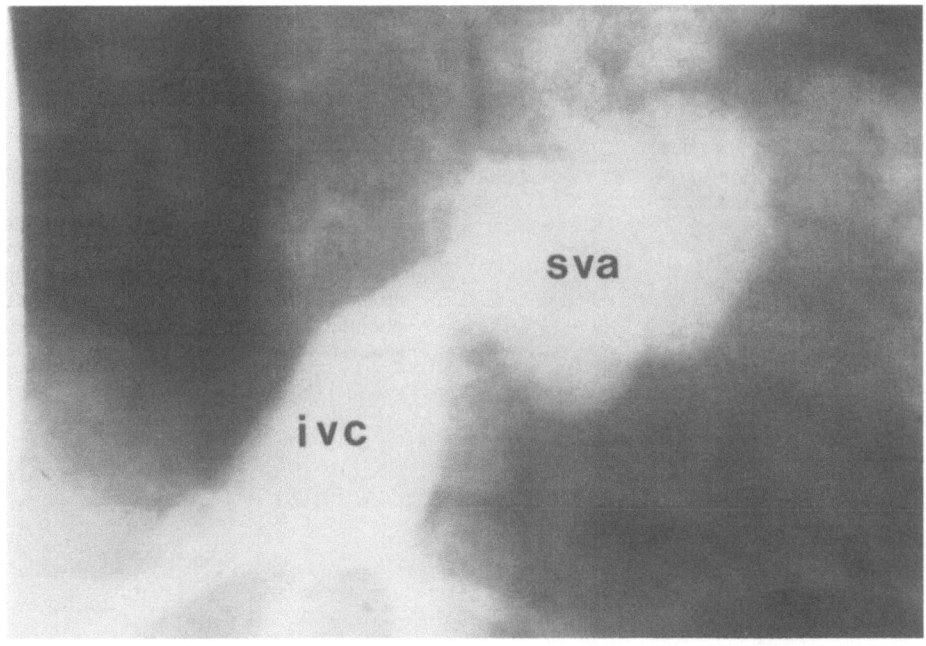

Fig. 1c. Angiocardiographic appearance after balloon dilatation shows much improved IVC pathway, although there is still some residual narrowing.

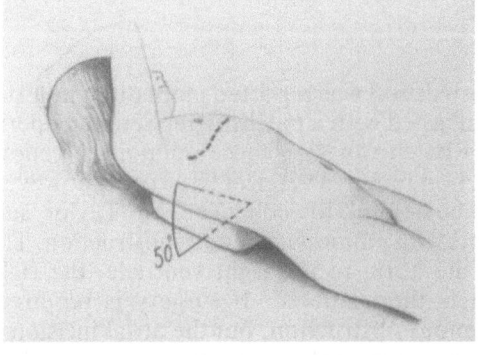

Fig. 2. Patient is positioned on the table with the right side elevated about 50°. The position of the thoracotomy is indicated by a dotted line.

sected and cannulated. Right atrium is opened from the right A-V groove to between the right pulmonary veins and the part of the old patch or even the whole baffle is removed. The new patch is tailored from a tube of Gore-tex of Dacron and adequate pathways are reconstructed (Fig. 3).

Pulmonary venous obstruction is less frequent but potentially a more serious complication. It may be caused by a wrong insertion of a Mustard baffle. If the suture line between the left and right pulmonary veins is parallel and does not diverge, obstruction may develop. Redundant baffle may also cause obstruction. It

139

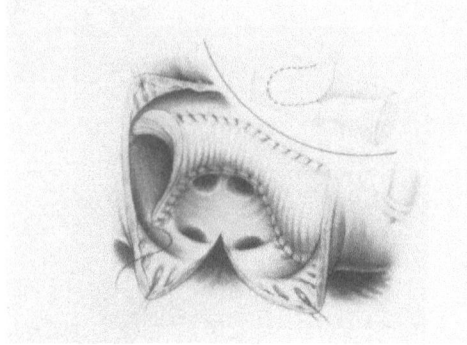

Fig. 3. The baffle has been removed and a new patch inserted. Note that the atrial incision runs deep to between the right upper and lower pulmonary vein. The patch is cut obliquely from a tube of Gore-tex or Dacron (insert).

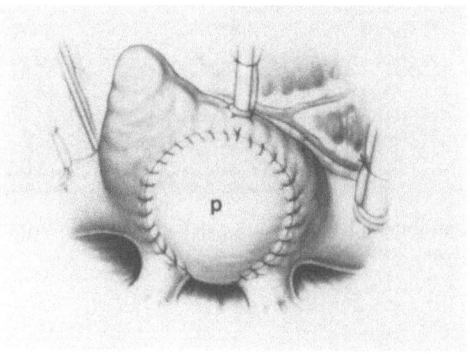

Fig. 4. Pulmonary venous atrium is opened across the obstruction into the posterior part of the atrium. Patch is then inserted to enlarge the pathway from the pulmonary veins towards the tricuspid valve. P – patch.

is of interest that pulmonary venous obstruction was reported more often in series where pulmonary venous atrium was enlarged with a patch. After Senning operation elongation of a septal flap with a patch can also cause pulmonary venous obstruction. Pulmonary venous obstruction requires surgical treatment, however, in some patients balloon dilatation may be helpful. My colleague, Dr. Taylor, successfully dilated three out of four patients with pulmonary venous obstruction. The balloon is passed retrograde through the aorta to the right ventricle, the right atrium and across the obstruction; it is then inflated. If surgery is required, approach is the same as for systemic venous obstruction, but the atrial incision is extended further behind into the posterior part of the pulmonary venous atrium and a patch, either of pericardium or Gore-tex is sewn in to separate the pulmonary veins and enlarge the pulmonary venous atrium (Fig. 4).

After atrial repair some patients are left with mild to moderate gradient from the left ventricle to the pulmonary artery, but only rarely does the obstruction progress. When the patient presents with suprasystemic pressure in the left ventricle treatment is indicated. The left-ventricular outflow tract obstruction is usually severe and in our experience is difficult to relieve. We approach this lesion from the left thoracotomy, cannulating the descending aorta and anatomical left atrium which, after Mustard or Senning operation, becomes systemic venous atrium. Left ventricular outflow tract obstruction is assessed from the pulmonary artery; if the

140

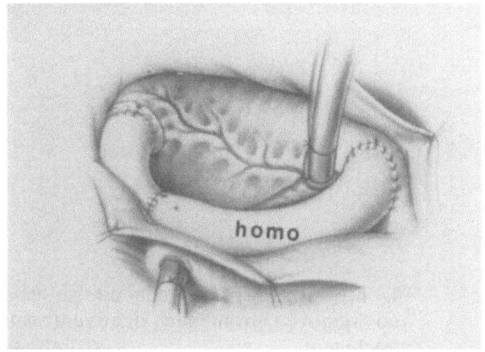

Fig. 5. Descending aorta is cannulated for arterial return and the left atrium, which, after atrial repair becomes systemic venous atrium, is used for the venous cannulation. A valved conduit is inserted between the apex of the left ventricle and the pulmonary artery. Homo − homograft.

lesion is resectable it is resected. If not, it is bypassed using LV to PA valved conduit [5] (Fig. 5).

Right-ventricular failure after atrial repair may be due to the fact that the right ventricle and the tricuspid valve are not suited to work as a systemic ventricle and a systemic AV valve. It may also be due to organic tricuspid valve incompetence or, perhaps, even to poor myocardial preservation at the original operation. The treatment can be either transplantation or we can use Dr. Mee's concept and change the Mustard or Senning operation into arterial switch after preliminary banding of the pulmonary artery [2].

Complications after anatomical repair

Complications may develop also after anatomical type of repair. After Rastelli operation, conduit obstruction, pulmonary artery branch stenoses, conduit or right-ventricular aneurysm, residual or recurrent VSD, left-ventricular outflow tract obstruction and residual/recurrent shunts were all observed. The performance of homografts in right-ventricular outflow tract depends on several factors. We have demonstrated earlier on that the length of the storage is important. Over 75% of homografts stored for less than 3 weeks in antibiotic solution were still functioning at 10 years. None of the homografts stored 3−6 weeks was functioning at 10 years. The current cryopreservation techniques will hopefully improve, if not solve, the problem of long-term homograft function. In addition, extension of a homograft with Dacron tube was also detrimental in our experience. Over 70% of homografts used alone or with a pericardial roof were functioning at 10 years, while only 40% of homografts extended with a Dacron tube were functioning at 10 years [5].

If the conduit becomes obstructed it has to be replaced. If it is firmly embedded in the posterior table of the sternum it may be safer to place the patient on iliac/iliac bypass before opening the sternum. The conduit is than transected and removed (Fig. 6). Pulmonary arteries are carefully inspected and any stenosis at the origin of the right or left pulmonary artery is repaired. The conduit is then replaced. Right-ventricular onflow tract is reconstructed either with the anterior cusp of the mitral valve of the homograft or a pericardial hood is attached to the homograft. The latter technique has to be used with a pulmonary homograft (Fig. 7). Alternatively,

141

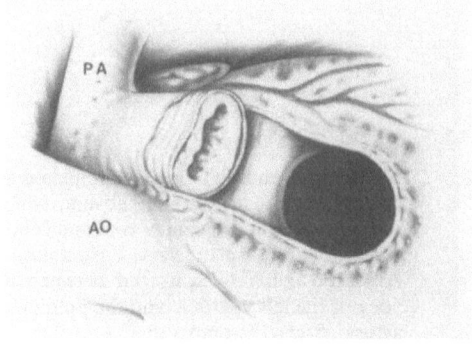

Fig. 6. Shows obstructed conduit transected and removed from the right-ventricular attachment.

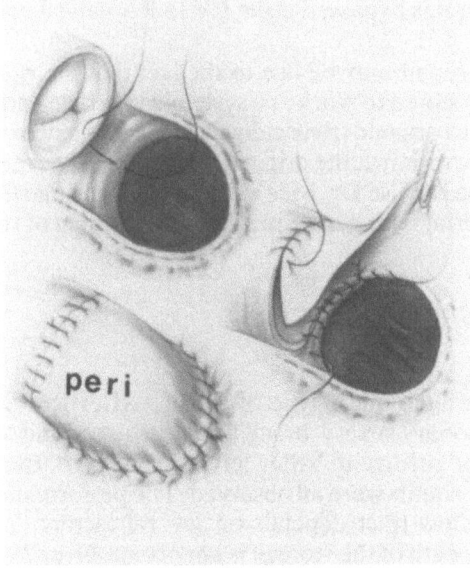

Fig. 7. Obstructed conduit is replaced with a new homograft. Peri − pericardial hood.

if a Dacron conduit had been used during the first operation the fibrous bed provides a good base for a tunnel which is completed with a pericardial or Gore-tex patch. This technique was described by Danielson [1].

Aneurysm or pseudoaneurysm of the right ventricle or a conduit can develop after Rastelli operation. Residual ventricular septal defect, infection or partial obstruction of the conduit are the main contributing factors. The lesion is approached either from the right thoracotomy or the patient is placed on femoro/femoral bypass and cooled before opening the sternum.

Left-ventricular outflow tract obstruction after Rastelli operation can be due to the narrowing at the previous VSD site, the whole tunnel may become small or the patient may develop subaortic shelf. Treatment is surgical. The roof of the left ventricle to aortic tunnel is approached through the right atrium or through the right

142

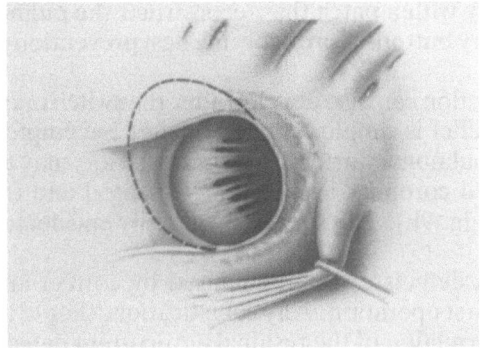

Fig. 8. Shows removal of the anterior portion of an LV to aorta tunnel. A small rim of the patch is left attached in the area of the conduction mechanism. Enlargement of the VSD is indicated by a dotted line.

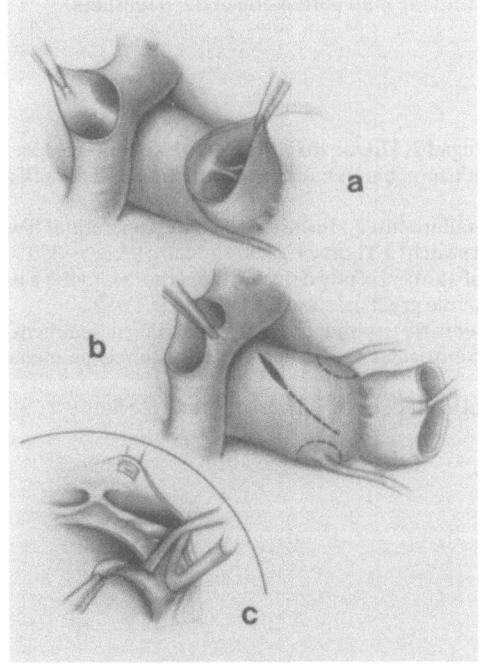

Fig. 9. Pulmonary artery is transected and the bifurcation retracted cephalad (Fig. 9a). Both transplanted coronaries are carefully identified and aortic root is opened (Fig. 9b). Subaortic fibrous shelf is ennucleated using a Watson Cheyne dissector (Fig. 9c).

ventricle and is opened. Most of the patch is removed, leaving only a rim in the area of the conduction system (Fig. 8). Ventricular septal defect is then enlarged in the lateral superior margin and a new tunnel is constructed. If the problem is due to subaortic shelf this is enucleated through the aortomy and aortic valve.

Complications were also described after arterial switch operation. A patient after this operation may develop right or left ventricular outflow tract obstruction, aortic valve incompetence or coronary artery stenosis or obstruction. Right ventricular outflow tract obstruction is usually at the level of the main pulmonary artery. It is relieved by longitudinal incision and insertion of a generous patch.

Elongation of the neopulmonary artery with a patch that reconstructs the pulmonary artery after removal of the coronary buttons is probably the best prevention of this complication.

Left-ventricular outflow tract obstruction can also develop after the switch operation. If it is a fibrous shelf, surgical relief is simple, but access after Lecompte's maneuvre may be difficult. The main pulmonary artery, which is anterior, may be transsected (Fig. 9a). The transplanted coronary arteries are visualised and the roof of the aorta is carefully opened (Fig. 9b). The shelf is then easily enucleated (Fig. 9c).

In conclusion, residual or recurrent defects can be minimised by correct and meticulous operative technique at the first operation. Any complications should be diagnosed early and accurately. The correction of the residual or recurrent defects is possible with a low risk if correct technique is used.

Acknowledgement: Figures 2−9 reproduced from "Reoperations in Cardiac Surgery" J. Stark and A. D. Pacifico (Eds.), Springer-Verlag (1989) with the kind permission of the publishers.

References

1. Danielson GK, Downing TP, Schaff HV, Puga FJ, DiDonato RM, Ritter DG (1987) Replacement of obstructed extracardiac conduits with autogenous tissue reconstructions. J Thorac Cardiovasc Surg 93:555−559
2. Mee RBB (1986) Severe right ventricular failure after Mustard or Senning operation. Two-stage repair: pulmonary artery banding and switch. J Thorac Cardiovasc Surg 92:385−390
3. Rashkind WJ, Miller WW (1966) Creation of an atrial septal defect without thoracotomy: a palliative approach to complete transposition of the great arteries. JAMA 196:991−992
4. Singh AK, Stark J, Taylor JFN (1976) Left ventricle to pulmonary artery conduit in treatment of transposition of great arteries, restrictive ventricular septal defect and acquired pulmonary atresia. Br Heart J 38:1213
5. Stark J (1989) Do we really correct congenital heart defects? J Thorac Cardiovasc Surg 97:1−9

Author's address:
J. Stark, MD FRCS
Cardiothoracic Unit
The Hospital for Sick Children
Great Ormond Street
London WC1N 3JH

Systolic and diastolic function after atrial repair of simple transposition of the great arteries

O. Reich, C. Ruth, M. Šamánek

Kardiocentrum. University Hospital Motol, Prague, Czechoslovakia

Introduction

In transposition of the great arteries the right ventricle is overloaded and its increased oxygen demands may not be met due to hypoxemia. During the surgery right-ventricular myocardium is exposed to an ischemic insult. After an atrial repair the volume overload is relieved, but the pressure overload persists. The overload, hypoxia, and ischemia may result in right-ventricular dysfunction. The disturbance in diastolic function may precede the systolic dysfunction [2]. Reported incidence of the right-ventricular dysfunction in simple transposition after an atrial repair ranges from 11 to 80 percent [4, 7−9, 12].

In our study, ventricular function in patients with an optimal result of an atrial repair of simple transposition was compared to right- and left-ventricular reference values derived from a group of children without any heart disease. Correlations were tested between the ventricular function parameters and preoperative pO_2, hemoglobin concentration, age at surgery, duration of the extracorporeal circulation and aortic cross-clamping time to evaluate a possible harmful effect of preoperative hypoxia and peroperative ischemia on the myocardium.

Methods

The radionuclide ventriculography was performed using Pho/Gamma LEM (Siemens) scintillation camera and PDP 11/34-Gamma 11 (DEC) System. ECG-gated blood pool scintigraphy was performed in left anterior oblique projection, providing optimal resolution of the ventricular septum. Five degrees detector caudal tilt and 30° slant-hole collimator were used for optimal atrio-ventricular separation. A total count of 8 million, 48 frames per cycle, and gate-tolerance of 10% of cycle duration were used. Ejection fractions were calculated from the background-free ventricular time-activity curves. The peak filling rates were computed as the maximal positive value of the first derivative of the ventricular time-activity curves; it was normalized for the end-diastolic volume (EDV/s). Reference values were derived from previously reported [11] results of 53 children who were subjected to a radionuclide shunt measurement (with subsequent radionuclide ventriculography) for suspected atrial septal defect and in whom the shunt was excluded. They were studied using the same protocol as in the transposition group. Mean values ± two standard deviations of the control group were considered the normal range.

Patients

Out of 76 patients studied after an atrial repair of simple transposition, 53 patients without residual defects were selected. In all, baffle leak, baffle obstruction, tricuspid regurgitation, and left-ventricular outflow tract obstruction were excluded by means of echocardiography and radionuclide angiocardiography. At the time of study, all were on sinus rhythm and in an excellent clinical condition. The Mustard procedure had been performed in 39 patients and the Senning procedure in 14 patients. The median age at surgery was 13 months with the range being from 1 months to 10.4 years. The median age at the study was 6.1 years, ranging from 19 months to 15.6 years. The median interval between the operation and the study was 4.7 years and ranged from 10 months to 10.9 years. Four patients had had a Blalock-Hanlon septectomy before the Mustard operation.

Results

There was no difference in ejection fractions between the patients and controls, either for the right or for the left ventricle (Fig. 1). The right-ventricular ejection fraction in transposition and control groups was equal (44 ± 6%). No patient had a right-ventricular ejection fraction below the normal range. The left-ventricular ejection fraction in the transposition group was 61 ± 7% as compared to 59 ± 6% in controls. One patient (1.9%) had a subnormal left-ventricular ejection fraction of 44% (normal range 47−71%).

The peak filling rates in the transposition group were nearly equal for both ventricles and significantly differed from both left- and right- ventricular references values (Fig. 2). Right- and left-ventricular peak filling rates were 2.50 ± 0.59 and 2.62 ± 0.77 EDV/s for the transposition group, as compared to 1.75 ± 0.43 and 3.11 ± 0.86 EDV/s for the controls.

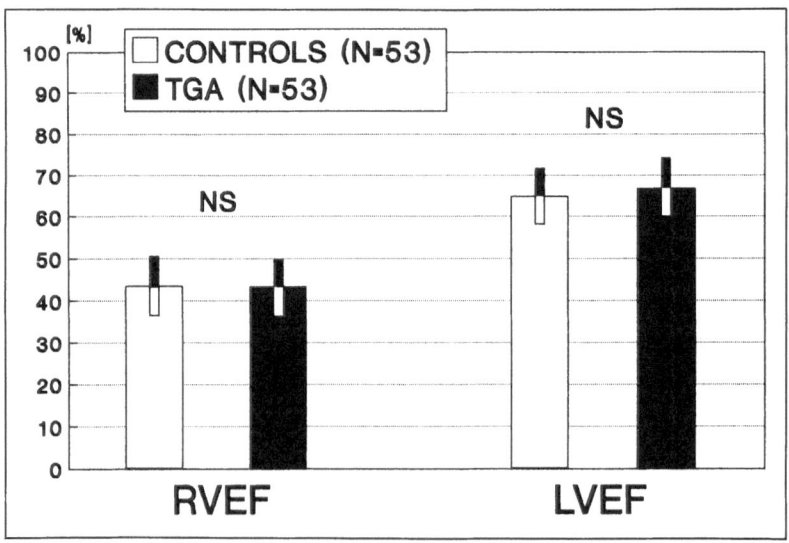

Fig. 1. Simple TGA after atrial repair ejection fractions

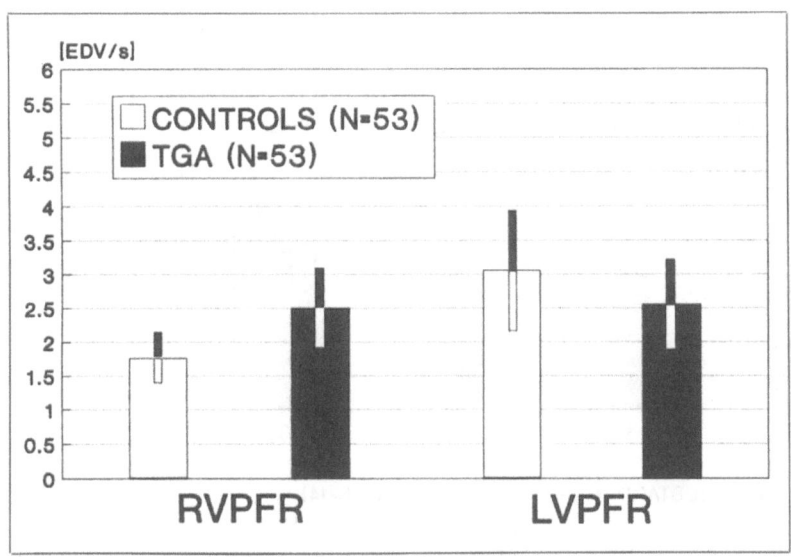

Fig. 2. Simple TGA after atrial repair peak filling rates

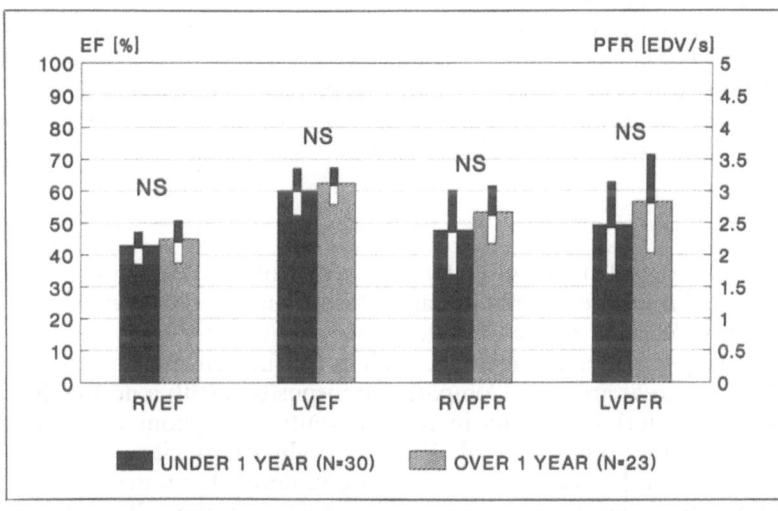

Fig. 3

There were weak negative correlations of the age at surgery (reflecting the duration of hypoxia) with the right-ventricular ejection fraction ($r = -0.34$, $p < 0.02$) and the right-ventricular peak filling rate ($r = -0.42$, $p < 0.002$). However, the decrease of the right-ventricular ejection fraction and the peak filling rate with increasing age at surgery was not steep enough to produce a significant difference between the patients operated in the first year of life and those operated later (Fig. 3). No correlation was found between the ventricular function parameters and preoperative pO_2, hemoglobin concentration, duration of the extracorporeal circulation, and aortic crossclamping time.

147

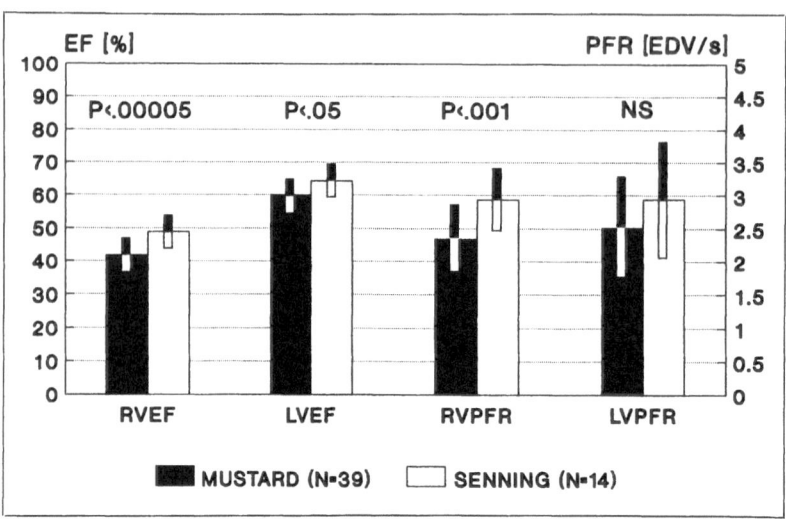

Fig. 4. Simple TGA after atrial repair according to the operation

After the Senning procedure all the parameters studied, except for the left-ventricular peak filling rate, were significantly higher than those after the Mustard procedure (Fig. 4). The respective values for Mustard and Senning groups were as follows: right-ventricular ejection fraction 41.5 ± 5 and $49 \pm 5\%$ ($p < 0.00005$), left-ventricular ejection fraction 60 ± 7 and $64 \pm 7\%$ ($p < 0.05$), right- ventricular peak filling rate 2.35 ± 0.56 and 2.94 ± 0.45 EDV/s ($p < 0.001$), left- ventricular peak filling rate 2.51 ± 0.73 and 2.94 ± 0.82 EDV/s (NS).

Discussion

Due to the methodological error caused by atrio-ventricular overlapping, parameters measured by radionuclide ventriculography differ from those measured by x-ray angiocardiography. Specific reference values must be used for each method. A controversy exists concerning the reference values for the ventricular function in transposition of the great arteries. Comparing transposition with a normal heart, reverse ventricular afterload results in reverse ventricular geometry [13] and reverse pressure-volume relations [10]. Elevated right-ventricular end-diastolic volume in transposition [1] may cause a decrease in derived parameters such as ejection fraction and filling rate. In our highly selective group, all the residual defects having influence on loading conditions such as regurgitation, shunt, and obstruction to inflow or outflow were excluded. The results of this group may perhaps be more suitable for comparison when studying ventricular function in transposition after the atrial repair than reference values for a normal heart. The independence of the parameters studied from preoperative hypoxia and perioperative ischemia of the myocardium supports this idea.

While the ejection fractions of both ventricles after the atrial repair of transposition did not differ from those in normal subjects, there was an important difference in ventricular peak filling rates. In absence of a semilunar valve regurgitation, the peak filling rate is influenced by capacity of atrial reservoir, pressure gradient across the AV valve and rate of ventricular relaxation. It correlates with maximal negative dP/dt, it is inversely related to ventricular end-diastolic pressure, but it is independent of passive diastolic properties such as modulus of chamber stiffness [5,7]. In our control group, the peak filling rate normalized for end-diastolic volume was independent of heart rate, age or body surface area [11]. Peak filling rates of both ventricles after the atrial repair of the transposition of the great arteries differ significantly from both control values. According to the obvious lack of difference between the right- and left-ventricular filling rates in the transposition group, we assumed that, rather than by the ventricular properties, the peak filling rates were influenced by the properties of the baffle. Also, the difference in filling between patients after the Mustard and Senning procedures may perhaps be explained by the different baffle properties [14].

In addition to the difference in diastolic function [1], better systolic function after the Senning procedure may be caused by a better myocardial protection in the Senning group operated later in our experience.

Conclusions

1) In simple transposition of the great arteries after an atrial repair without residual defects, the right and left ejection fractions are within normal limits.
2) Ventricular filling is abnormal for both ventricles, probably owing to the atrial baffle properties.
3) Ejection fractions and right-ventricular peak filling rates are higher after the Senning procedure than after the Mustard procedure.

References

1. Graham TP, Atwood GF, Boucek RJ, Boerth RC, Bender HW (1975) Abnormalities of right ventricular function following Mustard's operation for transposition of the great arteries. Circulation 52:678−674
2. Grossman W, Barry WH (1980) Diastolic pressure-volume relations in the diseased heart. Fed Proc 39:148−155
3. Hagler DJ, Ritter DG, Mair DD, Tajik AJ, Seward JB, Fulton RE, Ritman EL (1979) Right and left ventricular function after the Mustard Procedure in transposition of the great arteries. Am J Cardiol 44:276−283
4. Jarmakani MM, Canet RV (1974) Preoperative and postoperative right ventricular function in children with transposition of the great vessels. Circulation 49, 50(suppl II):39−45
5. Magorien DJ, Shaffer P, Bush C, Magorien RD, Kolibash AJ, Unverferth DV, Bashore TM (1984) Hemodynamic correlates for timing intervals, ejection rate and filling rate derived from the radionuclide angiocardiographic volume curve. Am J Cardiol 53:567−571
6. Miller TR, Grossman SJ, Schectman KB, Biello DR, Ludbrook PA, Ehsani AA (1986) Left ventricular diastolic filling and its association with age. Am J Cardiol 58:531−535
7. Murphy JH, Barlai-Kovach MM, Mathews RA, Beerman LB, Park SC, Neches WH, Zuberbuhler JR (1983) Rest and exercise right and left ventricular function late after Mustard operation: assessment by radionuclide ventriculography. Am J Cardiol 51:1520−1526
8. Ramsay JM, Venables AW, Kelly MJ, Kalff V (1984) Right and left ventricular function at rest and with exercise after the Mustard operation for transposition of the great arteries. Br Heart J 51:364−370
9. Redington AN, Rigby ML, Oldershaw P, Gibson DG, Shinebourne EA (1989) Right ventricular function 10 years after the Mustard operation for transposition of the great arteries: analysis of size, shape, and wall motion. Br Heart J 62:455−461

10. Redington AN, Rigby ML, Shinebourne EA, Oldershaw PJ (1990) Changes in the pressure-volume relation of the right ventricle when its loading conditions are modified. Br Heart J 63:45−49
11. Reich O, Krejcír M, Ruth C (1989) Results of radionuclide ventriculography in normal children and adolescents (in Czech). Cas Lek Ces 128:1321−1324
12. Trusler GA, Williams GA, Duncan KF, Hesslein PS, Benson LN, Freedom RM, Izukawa T, Olley PM (1987) Results with the Mustard operation in simple transposition of the great arteries 1963−1985. Ann Surg 206:251−260
13. Van Doesburg NH, Bierman FZ, Williams RG (1983) Left ventricular geometry in infants with d-transposition of the great arteries and intact ventricular septum. Circulation 68:733−739
14. Wyse RKH, Macartney FJ, Rohmer J, Ottenkamp J, Brom AG (1980) Differential atrial filling after Mustard and Senning repairs. Detection by transcutaneous Doppler ultrasound. Br Heart J 44:692−698

Author's address:
O. Reich, M.D.
Kardiocentrum
University Hospital Motol
V úvalu 84
CS-150 18, Prague
Czechoslovakia

P_{31} MR spectroscopy of right-ventricular myocardium after atrial repair for transposition of the great arteries

H. Stern, G. Schröter, K. Bühlmeyer

Arbeitsgruppe Kernspintomographie der TU München, Kinderkardiologie des Deutschen Herzzentrums München, FRG

Introduction

P_{31} MR spectroscopy (MRS) is a new noninvasive means which provides in vivo information about relative concentrations of myocardial high-energy phosphates and phospholipids in man. Phosphorus spectra of normal myocardium show different peaks for phosphocreatine (PCr), adenosine triphosphate (ATP), as well as for phosphodiesters (PDE) and phosphomonoesters (PME). Some of the resonances are contaminated by such compounds as NADP, NADPH or adenosindiphosphate, but these contributions usually account for less than 10% of the resonances. A typical example of a phosphorus spectrum for sceletal muscle is given in Fig. 1. As the various resonance peaks overlap, a mathematical curve fit has to be performed and is given as a dashed line in Fig. 1.

In animal studies as well as in a limited number of clinical studies, MRS has been performed in ventricular hypertrophy [5, 8], different forms of cardiomyopathy [5, 8, 14], and myocardial ischemia [13]. Changes in the myocardial composition of phospholipids have been reported both for ventricular hypertrophy and for some cardiomyopathies [6, 8]. In severely compromised myocardial function, PCr is usually reduced [3, 10].

In long-term observations of patients after atrial repair of transposition of the great arteries (TGA) late morbidity and mortality is evoked by arrhythmia and right-ventricular failure [12]. The reason for failure of the systemic right ventricle is, however, yet poorly understood. Differences in energy metabolism between normal left and hypertrophied right-ventricular myocardium may exert an unfavorable influence in these patients' long-term outcome.

Therefore, in this study it should be investigated if concentrations of high-energy phosphates and phospholipids, as assessed by MRS, in right-ventricular myocardium in patients after atrial repair for TGA are different from normal left-ventricular myocardium.

Methods

Patients

Twelve patients (mean age: 17.8 ± 1.9 years) after Mustard operation [4] for simple transposition of the great arteries were studied by MRS. The mean interval between surgery and MRS was 14.8 ± 1.9 years. Right-ventricular ejection fraction (RV-EF) was determined by multicycled and multisliced MR scans, as reported earlier [1]. Mean RV-EF was 51.9 (SD 7.8)% and was considered as normal in all patients.

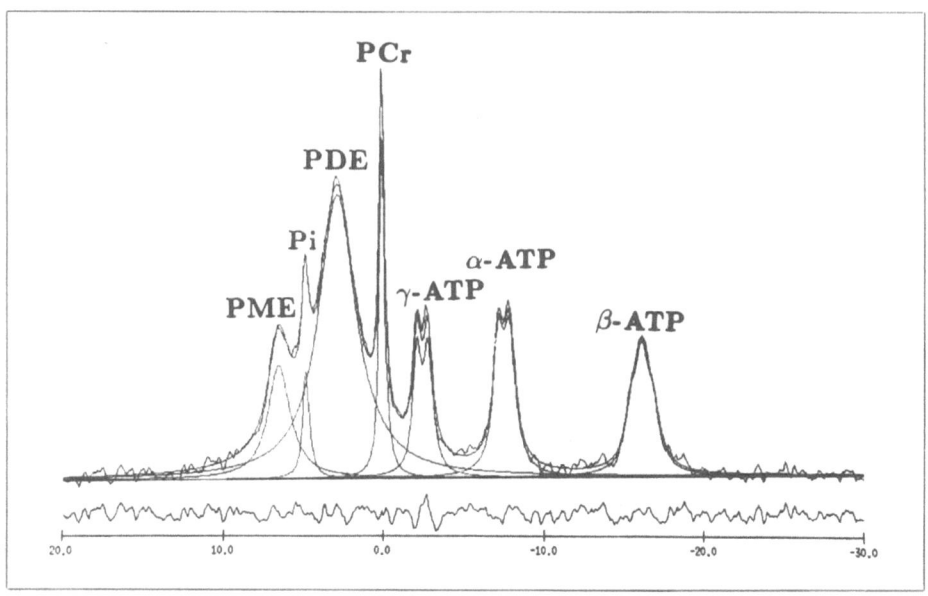

Fig. 1. Typical P31 spectrum of skeletal muscle in a healthy subject. Shown are resonance peaks for phosphocreatine (PCr), anorganic phosphor (Pi), phosphomonoesters and phosphodiesters, as well as for α-, β-, and γ-adenosine triphosphate (ATP). The upper lines represent original registrations, whereas the lower lines show mathematically fitted curves (see text).

Two control groups were investigated by MRS as well. One group comprised eight healthy volunteers with a mean age of 16.5 ± 2.8 years. The second control group consisted of six patients (mean age 14.8 ± 2.4 years) with compromised function of the systemic ventricle. Four of the six patients had dilative cardiomyopathy (dil-CMP) with a mean left-ventricular fraction shortening of 23.5 ± 2.7%, as assessed by m-mode echocardiography. Two patients had reduced right-ventricular function after Mustard operation for simple TGA. Right-ventricular EF in these patients was 42% and 31%, respectively.

P₃₁ MR Spectroscopy, data acquisition

MR spectra were obtained at 25.43 MHz using a commercially available imaging-spectroscopy system (Philips Gyroscan S15) working at 1.5 Tesla. The subjects lay prone on a 16-cm double-tuned surface coil. The center of the coil was positioned anterior to the free wall of the right ventricle in patients after Mustard operation and it was slightly rotated to the left for measurements in LV myocardium. Conventional proton MR images were acquired to confirm the location of the coil relative to the heart. In patients after atrial repair for TGA the sensitive volume was placed in the free wall of the right ventricle and interventricular septum. In healthy control subjects and in patients with dil-CMP the volume was located in the lateral wall of the left ventricle and interventricular septum. Mean size of the sensitive volume was 59 ± 14 ml and mean distance between the center of the coil and the vol-

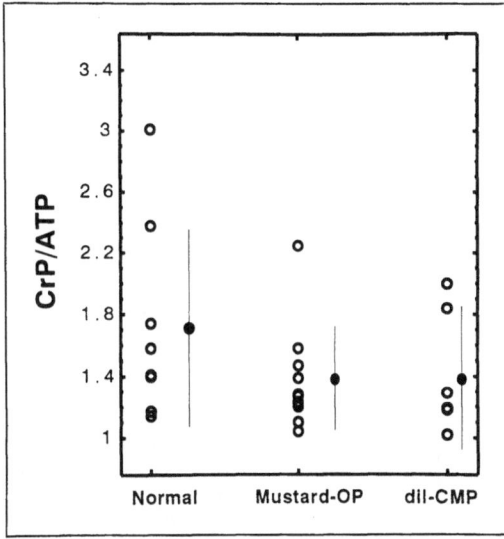

Fig. 2. Ratio of phosphocreatine (CrP) to adenosine triphosphate (ATP) in left- or right-ventricular myocardium in normal subjects as well as in patients with dilative cardiomyopathy (dil-CMP) or right-ventricular hypertrophy after Mustard operation.

ume was less than 8 cm. To minimize signal contamination by skeletal muscle the antero-posterior diameter of the volume was reduced to 25 mm.

Magnetic field homogeneity was optimized within the sensitive volume to 0.5–1.0 ppm by adjusting the field for narrowest tissue water resonance in H_1-spectra. For excitation of phosphorus compounds adiabatic pulses were used. The spectra acquisitions were ECG-triggered with the systolic cardiac phase and resulted from averaging 1024 free induction decays (FID) with an interpulse delay of 3 s. The entire investigation time ranged between 75–90 min.

Data analysis

Relative concentrations of myocardial phosphorus metabolites were measured from integrated areas under corresponding resonances. A Gauss filter equivalent to a line broadening of 20 Hz was applied to each FID to improve the signal to noise ratio of the resultant spectrum. The zero- and first-order phase corrections were applied. The resonances were fitted to Lorenzian lines, using a routine published previously [2]. From each data set relative concentrations of myocardial phosphorus metabolites were calculated by level ratios of PCr to the γ-peak ATP and phosphodiesters to ATP. The γ-peaks instead of the β-peaks were selected because of more reliable excitation [7]. Mean values of different phosphorus resonances were calculated for all study groups and tested for intergroup differences by unpaired Student's *t*-test.

Results

Individual and mean values for CrP/ATP and PDE/ATP are indicated in Figs. 2 and 3 for patients after atrial repair for TGA and for both control groups. No statis-

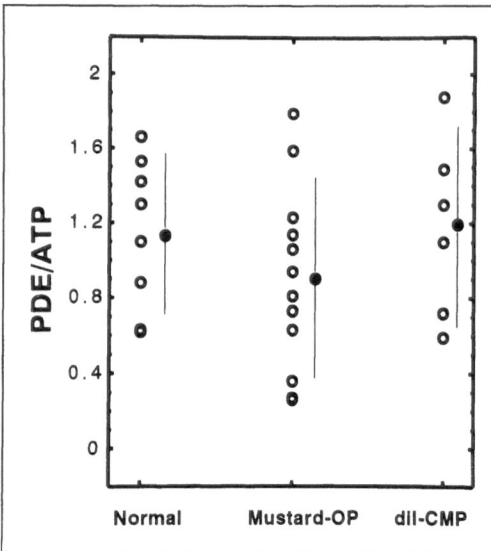

Fig. 3. Ratio of Phosphodiesters (PDE) to adenosine triphosphate (ATP) in left- or right-ventricular myocardium in normal subjects as well as in patients with dilative cardiomyopathy (dil-CMP) or right-ventricular hypertrophy after Mustard operation.

tically significant difference in relative concentrations of high-energy phosphates and phospholipids was observed in right-ventricular myocardium of patients after Mustard operation and normal left-ventricular myocardium. There was a tendency for a reduced CrP/ATP ratio and an elevated PDE/ATP ratio in patients with myocardial failure, compared to normals, but this difference did not gain statistical significance.

Comments

Decreased CrP/ATP ratios have been reported in two patients with hypertrophic cardiomyopathy [5], although most animal experiments reveal unchanged CrP and ATP concentrations in the hypertrophied myocardium [9, 11]. Schaefer et al. found no statistically significant changes of left-ventricular CrP/ATP ratio in patients with moderate or severe arterial hypertension [8]. In our series, patients after Mustard operation had CrP/ATP ratios in the hypertrophied RV myocardium which was not different from normal LV myocardium under resting conditions. From these data altered energy metabolism seems not to be a potential risk factor for right-ventricular failure after atrial repair for TGA. CrP/ATP ratios may change under exercise, as has been reported in patients with severe coronary artery stenosis [13], but MRS cannot be performed under exercise using present MR equipment. Our six patients with compromised ventricular function had a slightly reduced mean CrP/ATP value and elevated PDE/ATP ratio, but this was not statistically significant and proved not to be as marked as described by Schaefer et al. in a group of adult patients with dil-CMP or by Whitman in an infant with severe congenital dil-CMP [8, 14]. This may be due to the small number of investigated children in our series. Different etiologies in dilative cardiomyopathy probably also play a part in the only small changes of PDE/ATP and CrP/ATP ratios in our group of children with moderately compromised ventricular function.

References

1. Bauer R, v.d. Flierdt E, Busch U, Stettmeier H, Lutilsky L, Langer W, Allgayer B (1988) Quantifizierung der Herzfunktion mit der Kernspintomographie. Nukl Med 3:203−212
2. Burger C, McKinnon G, Buchli R, Boesiger P (1991) Towards fully automatic estimation of in vivo 31P spectra. Magn Res Med (in press)
3. Furchgott RF, Lee KS (1961) High energy phosphates and the force of contraction of cardiac muscle. Circulation 24:416−428
4. Mustard WT (1964) Successful two-stage correction of transposition of the great vessels. Surgery 55:469−472
5. Rajagopalan B, McKenna W, Blackledge M, Bolas N, Oberhänsli R, Radda GK (1988) Measurement of phosphorus metabolites in hearts of patients with hypertrophic cardiomyopathy by MRS (Abstract). Society of Magnetic Resonance in Medicine, Seventh Annual Meeting, San Francisco 1:296
6. Reibel DK, O'Rourke B, Foster KA, Hutchinson H, Uboh CE, Kent RL (1986) Altered phospholipid metabolism in pressure-overloaded hypertrophied hearts. Am J Physiol 250:H1−H6
7. Schaefer S, Gober J, Valenza M, Karczmar GS, Matson GB, Camacho SA, Botvinick EH, Massie B, Weiner MW (1988) Nuclear magnetic resonance imaging-guided Phosphorus-31 spectroscopy of the human heart. JACC 12:1449−1455
8. Schaefer S, Gober JR, Schwartz GC, Twieg DB, Weiner MW, Massie B (1990) In vivo Phosphorus-31 spectroscopic imaging in patients with global myocardial disease. Am J Cardiol 65:1154−1161
9. Shimamoto N, Goto N, Tanabe M, Imamoto T, Fujiwara S, Hirata M (1982) Myocardial energy metabolism in the hypertrophied heart of spontaneously hypertensive rats. Basic Res Cardiol 77:359−367
10. Swain JL, Sabina RL, Peyton RB, Jones RN, Wechsler AS, Holmes EW (1982) Derangements in myocardial purine and pyrimidine nucleotide metabolism in patients with coronary artery disease and left ventricular hypertrophy. Proc Natl Acad Sci USA 79:655−659
11. Tubau JF, Wikman-Coffelt J, Massie BM, Sievers R, Parmley WW (1987) Improved myocardial efficiency in the working perfused heart of the SHR. Hypertension 10:396−403
12. Turina MI, Siebenmann R, v. Segesser L, Schönbeck M, Senning A (1989) Late functional deterioration after atrial correction for transposition of the great arteries. Circulation 80 (suppl II):I162−I167
13. Weiss RG, Bottomley PA, Hardy CJ, Gerstenblith G (1990) Regional myocardial metabolism of high-energy phosphates during isometric exercise in patients with coronary artery disease. New Engl J Med 1990:1593−1600
14. Whitman GJR, Chance BC, Bode H, Maris J, Haselgrove J, Kelley R, Clark BJ, Harken AH (1985) Diagnosis and therapeutic evaluation of a pediatric case of cardiomyopathy using Phosphorus-31 nuclear magnetic resonance spectroscopy. JACC 5:745−749

Author's address:
Dr. Heiko Stern
Deutsches Herzzentrum München
− Kinderkardiologie −
Lothstraße 11
D-8000 München 2
FRG

Supra pulmonary stenosis after arterial switch operation for transposition of the great arteries

E. J. Meijboom, J. Punt, R. P. Beekman, P. A. Hutter, W. J. L. Suijker,
H. J. C. M. van de Wal, E. Harinck
Department of Pediatric Cardiology, Wilhelmina Children's Hospital, University
of Utrecht, Utrecht, The Netherlands

Introduction

Up until 25 years ago, the mortality rate of untreated transposition of the great arteries was about 90% during the first year of life. The Rashkind balloon atrio-septostomy [5], introduced in 1966, increased effective flow in both circulations and, therefore, diminished cyanosis. This decrease in cyanosis was associated with a significant decrease in the mortality rate. However, the blood exchange at atrial level does not keep up with the increasing flow dimension of children during growth. The Mustard operation, which establishes an atrial switch [4] was developed, and proved to have a low operative mortality rate; it also allows a total separation of pulmonary and systemic circulation. The atrial switch remained, therefore, the operation of choice in the following two decades. Initial enthusiasm for this operation, however, subsided when complications such as obstruction of the venous pathways, arrhythmias, and right-ventricular dysfunction caused a staggering increase in late mortality. The development of the arterial switch operation [1] suggested a new surgical treatment for patients with transposition of the great arteries without the previously stated severe complications.

At the Wilhelmina Children's Hospital, we therefore changed our operating technique and started to perform the arterial switch operation since 1977. Initially, we used the Jatene technique until 1982; thereafter the Lecompte technique [2] was preferred. In order to evaluate our degree of success, we studied 85 patients after arterial switch operation and found none of the previous mentioned complications of the atrial switch, but encountered obstruction or stenosis of the pulmonary system as the major residual problem.

Type of operation

Starting in 1977, the Jatene-type of arterial switch operation was employed in the Wilhelmina Children's Hospital in order to prevent venous obstruction, arrhythmias, and right-ventricular dysfunction as complications. In the inital phase a two-stage operation was performed, including an initial banding of the main pulmonary artery in order to adjust left-ventricular performance, sometimes combined with the establishment of an aorto-pulmonary shunt. The second stage of the operation was the actual arterial switch operation, with debanding of the pulmonary artery and closure of the aorto-pulmonary shunt (in some cases a graft was interposed in the main pulmonary artery and, in one case, in the ascending aorta). Since 1982, the two-stage operation was abandoned and immediate arterial switching was performed on patients with transposition of the great arteries within the first week of life. Starting in 1982, the Lecompte manuever was employed on most of the patients, except for those patients with a predominantly side-by-side position of the great arteries.

Materials and methods

Eighty-five patients after arterial switch of the great arteries (1977 to 1991) were followed. Patients were followed on an out-patient clinic basis with yearly intervals. The investigations included a general physical examination, auscultation of the heart, ECG and two-dimensional (2D) Doppler echocardiographic evaluation. Special care was given to the imaging and obtaining of flow velocities of the right-ventricular outflow tract and pulmonary arteries. MRI studies and cardiac catheterization were performed when the presence of significant pulmonary stenosis was suspected.

Results

Out of 85 patients, 64 were "switched" using the Lecompte technique. Twenty-one patients were switched according to the Jatene technique; five of these had an interposition of a patch in the pulmonary artery; and one in the aorta (Fig. 1).

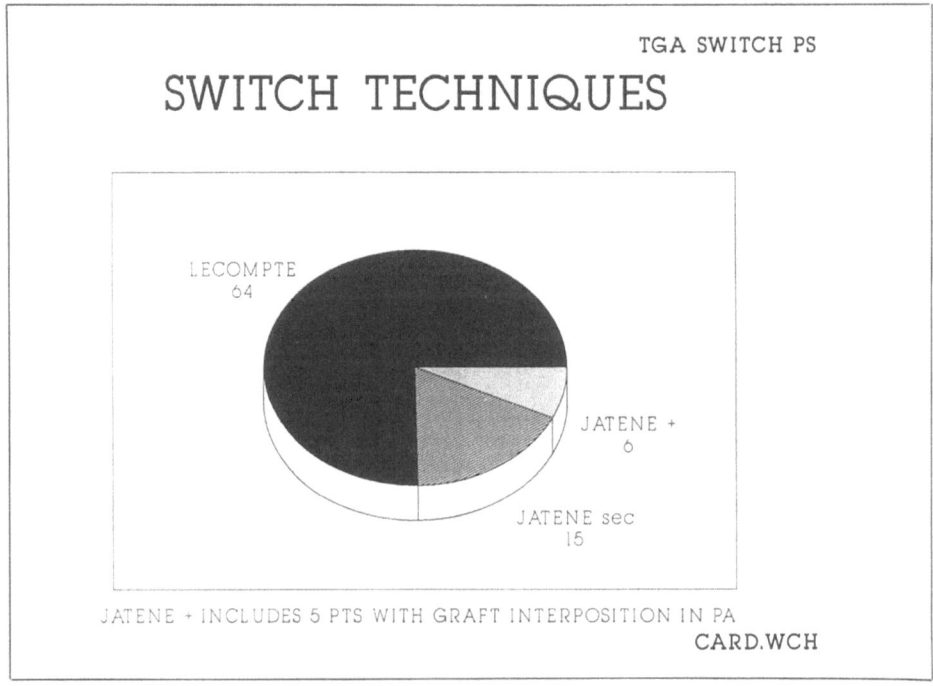

Fig. 1. The group of 85 patients with TGA. Divided according to the arterial switch technique used.

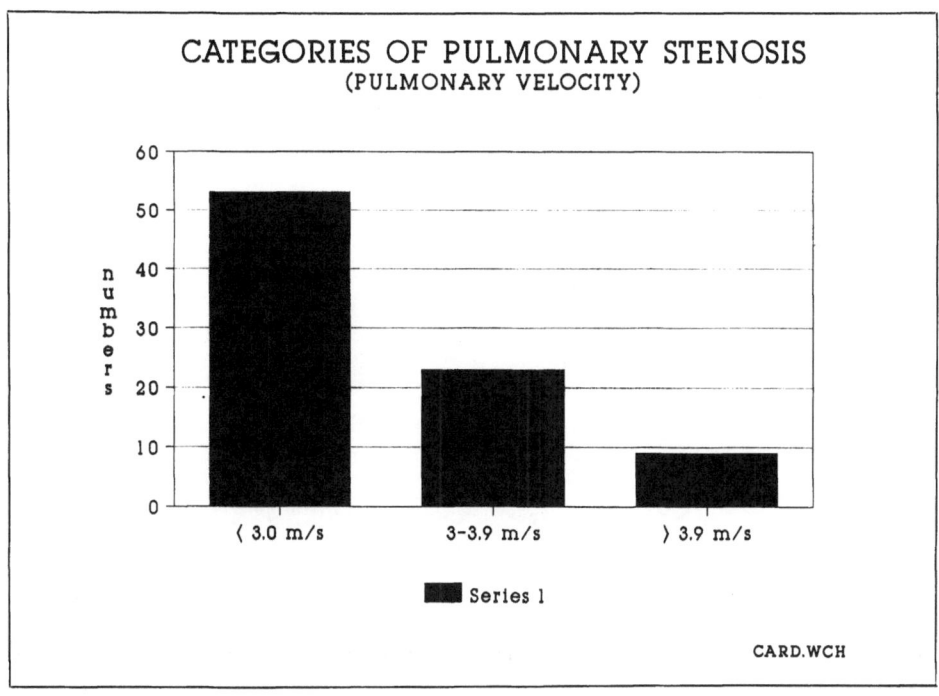

Fig. 2. The pulmonary flow velocities measured in all patients.

The spectrum of flow velocities encountered by 2D-echocardiography varies from 0.6 to 5 m/s (Fig. 2). Pulmonary stenosis (flow velocity over 3 m/s) was encountered in 38% of our population (n = 32); 27% had a mild to moderate stenosis (3–3.9 m/s), 10% had severe stenosis (>4 m/s).

Comparing the severity of the pulmonary stenosis per switch technique used, no significant differences between these two switch techniques were encountered (Fig. 3). 57% of the patients of the Jatene group had no pulmonary stenosis, 33% appeared to have a mild to moderate pulmonary stenosis; 10%, however, suffered from a severe pulmonary stenosis. In the Lecompte group 64% had no sign of pulmonary stenosis, 25% had a mild to moderate pulmonary stenosis, 11% suffered from a severe pulmonary stenosis.

Localization of the pulmonary stenosis is either in the pulmonary truncus (n = 20), the pulmonary branches (n = 10), or it could not be localized on 2D-echocardiography (n = 2). One pulmonary branch stenosis was encountered after using the Jatene technique (11% of pulmonary stenoses in this group). Pulmonary branch stenoses after using the Lecompte technique, however, was encountered in nine patients (39% of pulmonary stenoses in this group) (Fig. 4). Pulmonary trunk stenosis was encountered in 78% of the pulmonary stenoses after the switch according to the Jatene technique, and in 57% of the pulmonary stenoses after the switch according to the Lecompte technique.

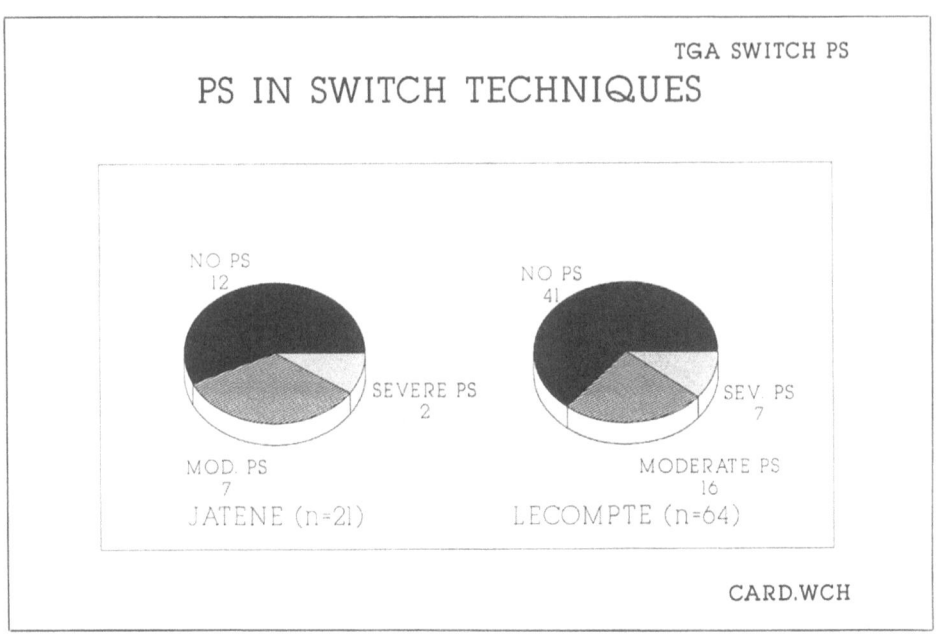

Fig. 3. The severity of pulmonary stenosis. The patients are divided according to the arterial switch technique used.

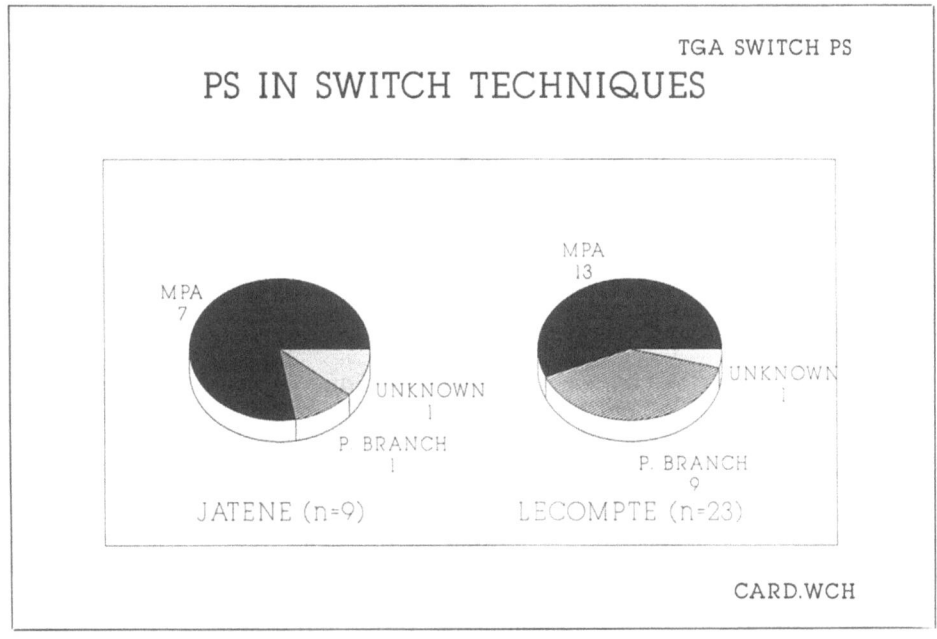

Fig. 4. The group of patients with a pulmonary stenosis (v > 3 m/s). Localization is either in the main pulmonary artery (MPA), in the pulmonary branch, or it could not be diagnosed.

Discussion

It can be concluded from our results that arterial inversion can be succesfully performed in complete transposition at the neonatal age. In all our patients a Rashkind procedure has been carried out preceeding surgery. The previously stated complications of the atrial switch operation arrhythmias, venous obstruction, and right-ventricular dysfunction have not occurred in our group. The only major complication we encountered was pulmonary stenosis in the newly created pulmonary artery trunk and in its branches, as described previously by Yacoub [3]. This late type of complication occurred in 38% of our operated patients. A large majority of these, however, shows a mild to moderate obstruction which does not impose any serious problems for the patients. The pulmonary stenosis can be divided into pulmonary artery trunk stenoses and pulmonary artery branch stenoses.

Pulmonary artery trunk stenosis occurs both in the Jatene-type of arterial switch and in the Lecompte-type of arterial switch, and is generally located at the site of the anastomosis. This location of the pulmonary stenosis is generally accessible for balloon dilatation of the stenosis, which in our group has been performed so far in three patients. Only one of these dilatations was succesful, the failures in the other two dilatations were caused by the location of the stenosis. Differing from pulmonary valve stenosis, where dilatation is generally succesful, this type of trunk stenosis is located relatively close to the bifurcation of the pulmonary artery, thus preventing optimal positioning of the balloon catheter.

The second type of pulmonary stenosis is the stenosis of pulmonary artery branches. This type stenosis is almost exclusively encountered in patients after the Lecompte procedure. The only patient with Jatene procedure in this category had a unilateral pulmonary artery stenosis, secondary to aortic compression. The group of patients with pulmonary branch stenosis after the Lecompte procedure generally had stenoses of both pulmonary artery branches located immediately after the bifurcation and lateral to the aorta. This type of pulmonary stenosis is usually inaccessible for balloon dilatation.

The pathophysiology of this stenosis can be secondary, due to inadequate operative mobilization of the pulmonary artery branches. However, being aware of this problem, the utmost care was taken to mobilize the pulmonary arteries right into the hilus.

A disturbed vascularization of the pulmonary artery branches after surgery is also suggested for this type of stenosis. The most likely explanation, however, is the stretching phenomen caused by the mobilization of the main pulmonary artery on the anterior side of the aorta and the stretching of the branches alongside the aorta into the hilus. The precise localization of the pulmonary stenosis is frequently difficult or impossible to obtain by 2-D Doppler echocardiography.

We can conclude that the diagnosis of this type of post-operative problem can be facilitated by the use of MRI imaging, as shown in our study. Based on the MRI results, patients were selected for further invasive diagnostic procedures, such as cardiac catheterization.

We remain in favor of the arterial switch repair of simple as well as complex transposition, despite the existence of complications as mentioned above. Specifically, when care is taken to free the pulmonary branches and to prevent trunk stenosis. However, until the long-term follow-up of our patients into adolescence and adulthood has been completed, we need to reserve our enthusiasm.

References

1. Jatene AD, Fontes VF, Paulista PP et al. (1976) Anatomic correction of transposition of the great vessels. J Thorac Cardiovasc Surg 72:364
2. Lecompte Y, Zannini L, Hazan E et al. (1981) Anatomic correction of transposition of the great arteries: new technique without use of a prosthetic conduit. J Thorac Cardiovasc Surg 82:629
3. Martin RP, Ladusans EG, Parsons JM et al. (1988) Incidence and site of pulmonary stenosis after anatomical correction of TGA. Br Heart J 59:122
4. Mustard WT (1964) Succesful two-stage correction of transposition of the great vessels. Surgery 55:469
5. Rashkind WJ, Miller WW (1966) Creation of an atrial septal defect without thoracotomy. JAMA 196:991

Authors' address:
Dr. E. J. Meijboom
Department of Pediatric Cardiology
Wilhelmina Children's Hospital
University of Utrecht
Utrecht
The Netherlands

The role of myocardial perfusion scintigraphy and echocardiographic wall-motion analysis in the postoperative assessment of patients after the arterial-switch operation

M. Vogel, H. Meisner*, J. F. Smallhorn**, K. Bühlmeyer
Department Pediatric Cardiology and Cardiac Surgery*, German Heart Center, Munich, FRG
** Hospital for Sick Children, Toronto, Canada

Introduction

One of the concerns about the results of the arterial switch operation is the adequacy of coronary artery perfusion. It may be compromised by coronary ostial stenosis or kinking following coronary artery reimplantation [3]. Anecdotal reports have revealed occassional myocardial infarction and unexplained sudden cardiac deaths [1, 10] with necropsy confirmation of myocardial infarction in one of these cases [12]. A simple noninvasive reproducible method of assessing integrity of myocardial perfusion in patients with transposition after the arterial switch operation is desirable. Unfortunately, the easiest method, the surface electrocardiogram is not very reliable, as a normal tracing at rest does not rule out myocardial ischemia [9, 14]. Other noninvasive methods include thallium myocardial perfusion scans [2] and echocardiographic analysis of regional left-ventricular wall motion [11], which were used in this study to address the problem of adequacy of myocardial blood supply after the arterial switch operation.

Methods

Thallium perfusion scintigraphy

The first part of the study involved patients from the Hospital for Sick Children in Toronto, who underwent a thallium perfusion scan with tomographic imaging using single photon emission computed tomography (SPECT) [5, 16]. This SPECT study was considered the gold standard of myocardial perfusion defect detection to which echocardiography was compared. Details of the thallium myocardial perfusion scan study have been published elsewhere [20]. Briefly, 21 patients, among them 14 after a two-stage anatomic correction following previous pulmonary artery banding, and seven newborns with primary switch operation were studied. Isoproterenol was used to simulate stress. During isoproterenol infusion heart rate increased from a mean 89 ± 15 to 135 ± 22 beats/min. At maximal heart rate a dose of 1.5-4 MBq/kg body weight ^{201}Tl was injected and imaging began with a General Electric 400 AC Starcam tomographic camera. The camera was rotated clockwise in a 180° arc to acquire 64 raw data images. Redistribution tomographic images were similarily obtained 2.5 h post injection and were considered to represent the resting phase. The scans were independently reviewed by two experienced reviewers.

Irreversible perfusion defects, which are present at isoproterenol-induced stress and during reperfusion represent myocardial infarction [2], while defects present at stress, but absent at reperfusion point to a problem with coronary artery flow reserve [6].

Echocardiography

Imaging was performed with commercially available equipment consisting of an ATL (Advanced Technology Laboratories) Ultramark eight- or nine-sector scanner. Wall-motion analysis was performed using an off-line computer system. The standard parasternal short-axis view and the apical four-chamber view were used for wall-motion analysis. In the parasternal short-axis view this was evaluated at the mitral valve, papillary muscle, and apical level. In newborns, we also used the subcostal four-chamber view and a subcostal short-axis view, in addition to the ones mentioned above. End-diastolic and end-systolic frames were selected as the ones showing the largest and smallest left-ventricular cross-sectional areas, respectively. The endocardial borders of these frames were digitized by hand through the use of a light pen connected to a digitizing tablet that was interfaced with a TV monitor. An enddiastolic and endsystolic frame were planimetered separately. Following that, the center of mass was calculated for each frame using a previously published formula [17]. A reference line was drawn connecting the center of mass with an outside reference point presented by the junction of the septal tricuspid leaflet with the interventricular septum. The centers of mass of the diastolic and systolic frames were superimposed and the reference lines aligned to correct for translation and rotation of the heart (floating system). The figure was then divided into eight equal radial segments starting in a clockwise fashion from the reference line. The regional area change for each segment was measured as ((diastolic area − systolic area): diastolic area) × 100. A previously described left-ventricular segmental system was used [8] for appropriate spatial nomenclature of the individual segments at mitral valve (basal segments), papillary muscle (midventricular segments), and apical level. The reproducibility of the regional left-ventricular wall-motion measurements has previously been assessed by analysis of intra- and interobserver variability, and we have published normal data for different age groups [18]. Global left-ventricular function was assessed by measuring endocardial enddiastolic and endsystolic volume using a modified Simpsons rule [15] from the apical two- and four-chamber view and calculating global ejection fraction as ((diastolic volume − systolic volume): diastolic volume) × 100. These data were compared with normal values previously established from our echocardiographic laboratory [18].

Patient selection

For the Toronto study, we selected 21 out of 46 survivors of an arterial-switch operation, who had come from within 100 kms of the city of Toronto and had agreed to participate in the study. For the second part of the study. we selected 60 consecutive patients with transposition of the great arteries and intact ventricular septum, who had undergone the arterial-switch operation as newborns at a mean age of 10 days during a period ranging from August 1987 to April 1991 at the German Heart

Table 1. Perfusion defects and echocardiographic wall-motion abnormalities after arterial-switch operation

Echocardiographic wall-motion abnormality	Perfusion defect	Anatomical location
Anterolateral wall	Irreversible	Anterolateral wall and apex
Apex	Irreversible	Apex
Apex	Irreversible	Apex
Septum	irreversible	Interventricular septum
Apex	Reversible	Apex
Anterolateral wall	Reversible	Inferolateral wall and apex
Apex	Reversible	Apex
None	Reversible	Basilar septum

Center in Munich. Those newborns had undergone a wall-motion analysis 1−2 days before surgery and a mean 20 days as well as 3 and 6 months after arterial switch operation. In those patients, left-ventricular enddiastolic volume and mass as well as ejection fraction have also been determined.

Results

Thallium scintigraphy

Table 1 lists the results of the thallium myocardial perfusion scintigraphy and concomitant echocardiographic wall-motion studies in the 21 patients in Toronto. Perfusion defects and wall-motion abnormalities were only found in those patients who had undergone a two-stage operation after prior pulmonary artery banding. In two of those patients aortography revealed a narrowed origin of the left coronary artery. One patient with a perfusion defect in the area of the basilar septum had a normal regional wall motion and normal global function, whereas in the remaining seven patients there was a wall-motion abnormality in a corresponding anatomic segment of the left ventricle, in which the perfusion was abnormal. Using thallium scintigraphy as a gold standard, the sensitivity of echocardiographic wall-motion analysis to detect myocardial perfusion defects is 87%, while the specificity is 100%.

Echocardiography

The echocardiographic wall-motion study in the 60 newborns in Munich had been normal in all before the arterial-switch operation. Figure 1 shows the regional left-ventricular wall motion in the 60 newborns examined before surgical intervention. Postoperatively, wall-motion abnormalities were present in three of the 60 newborns. These abnormalities could be detected at all three follow-up examinations. In one patient they were detected in the segments representing the anterolateral wall and the apex, in the second patient they were present in the anterolateral wall, and in the third patient in the area of the basilar septum. The aortic root angiogram

165

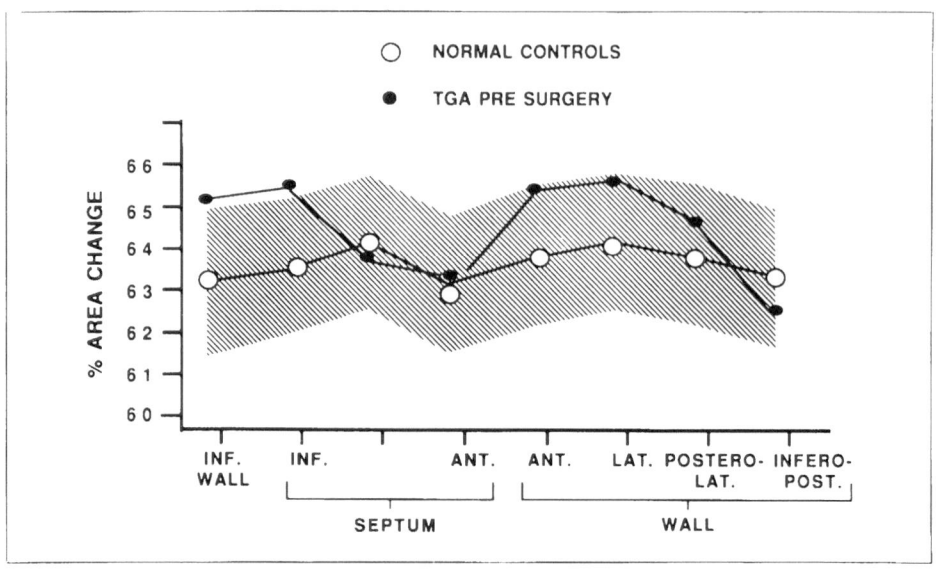

Fig. 1. Left-ventricular wall motion at papillary muscles level before arterial-switch operation in 60 newborns and 15 controls.

in the first patient with the wall-motion abnormalities is shown in Dr. Sauer's contribution to this volume, and it reveals retrograde filling of the left coronary artery, which was occluded at its origin. Figure 2 shows the wall motion abnormality in the second patient with the reduced area change in the segments representing the anterolateral wall. In Figs. 3a and 3b the pre- and postoperative electrocardiogram's of the same patient are shown. There is marked decrease of R-wave in the left precordial leads with ST-depression and T-wave changes. Global left-ventricular ejection fraction was 72% in all newborns before surgery, 67% 5 days post surgery, and 72% 3 months post surgical repair of transposition. The left- ventricular volume at the last examination was within the normal range of our controls in all patients. Figure 4 shows the graphic display of left-ventricular volume in the normal controls and those patients who did not have evidence of wall-motion abnormalities. It demonstrates normal LV volume present in all patients with normal regional wall motion. The overall incidence of persistent wall motion abnormalities was 5%.

Discussion

Myocardial ischemia after arterial-switch operation

Although the incidence of impairment of myocardial perfusion is low in the studies published about the intermediate follow-up of the arterial switch operation [10, 12, 21], myocardial ischemia is associated with a potentially high morbidity [1] and even mortality [3, 12]. In addition, wall-motion abnormalities detected invasively by angiography were found in 7 of 17 patients after the arterial switch operation [7].

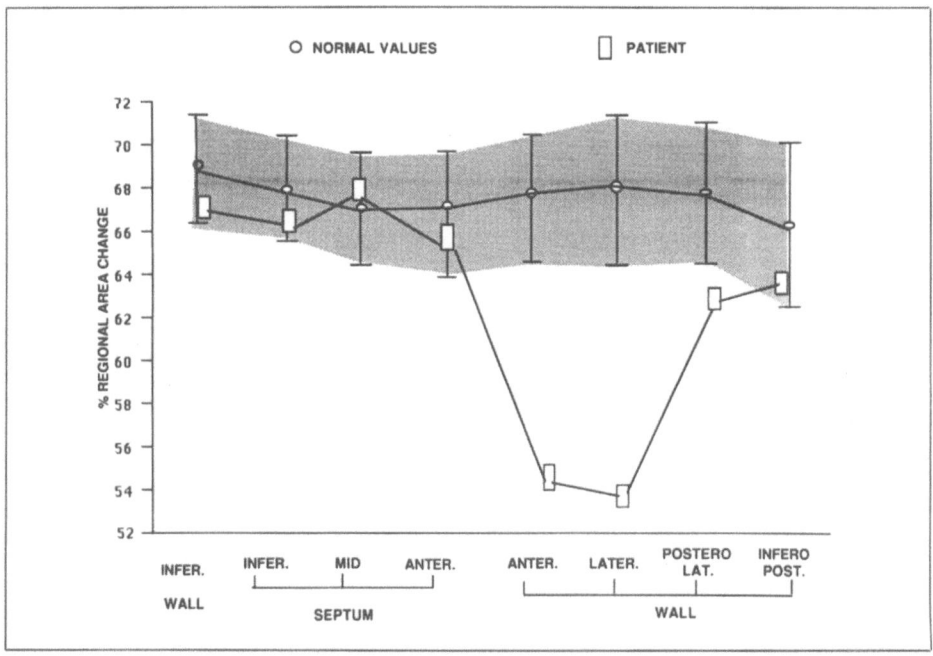

Fig. 2. Left-ventricular wall motion at papillary muscles level after arterial switch in the second patient with a wall-motion abnormality.

A reliable noninvasive diagnostic method to detect myocardial ischemia is desirable. The surface electrocardiogram may not be sensitive enough [9] to detect myocardial infarction. In addition, the majority of the patients with transposition and intact ventricular septum in both studies had an incomplete bundle branch block, which makes detection of signs of myocardial ischemia even more difficult.

Thallium scintigraphy

Thallium myocardial perfusion scintigraphy has been extensively evaluated in adult patients, both with normal hearts and with proven coronary artery disease [4, 16]. Some normal subjects were found to have regional heterogeneity in the basal segments of the heart, but otherwise, the incidence of false-positive findings was low [4]. Overall, the sensitivity of thallium perfusion scintigraphy to detect myocardial ischemia is close to 95% (and specificity in one study was 92% [16]), if both initial and redistribution imaging is used and if a SPECT study is performed [2, 4]). These two latter technical requirements had been fulfilled in our study. One significant problem of thallium myocardial perfusion scintigraphy is the amount of irradiation, especially to the gonads, as thallium is excreted via the kidneys and radioactivity may persist in the bladder for more than 24 h [5]. This may limit its applicability in newborns and young children. Because of the high dose of radiation to the gonads, we would currently not recommend routine use of thallium myocardial perfusion scans in assymptomatic newborns after the arterial-switch operation.

167

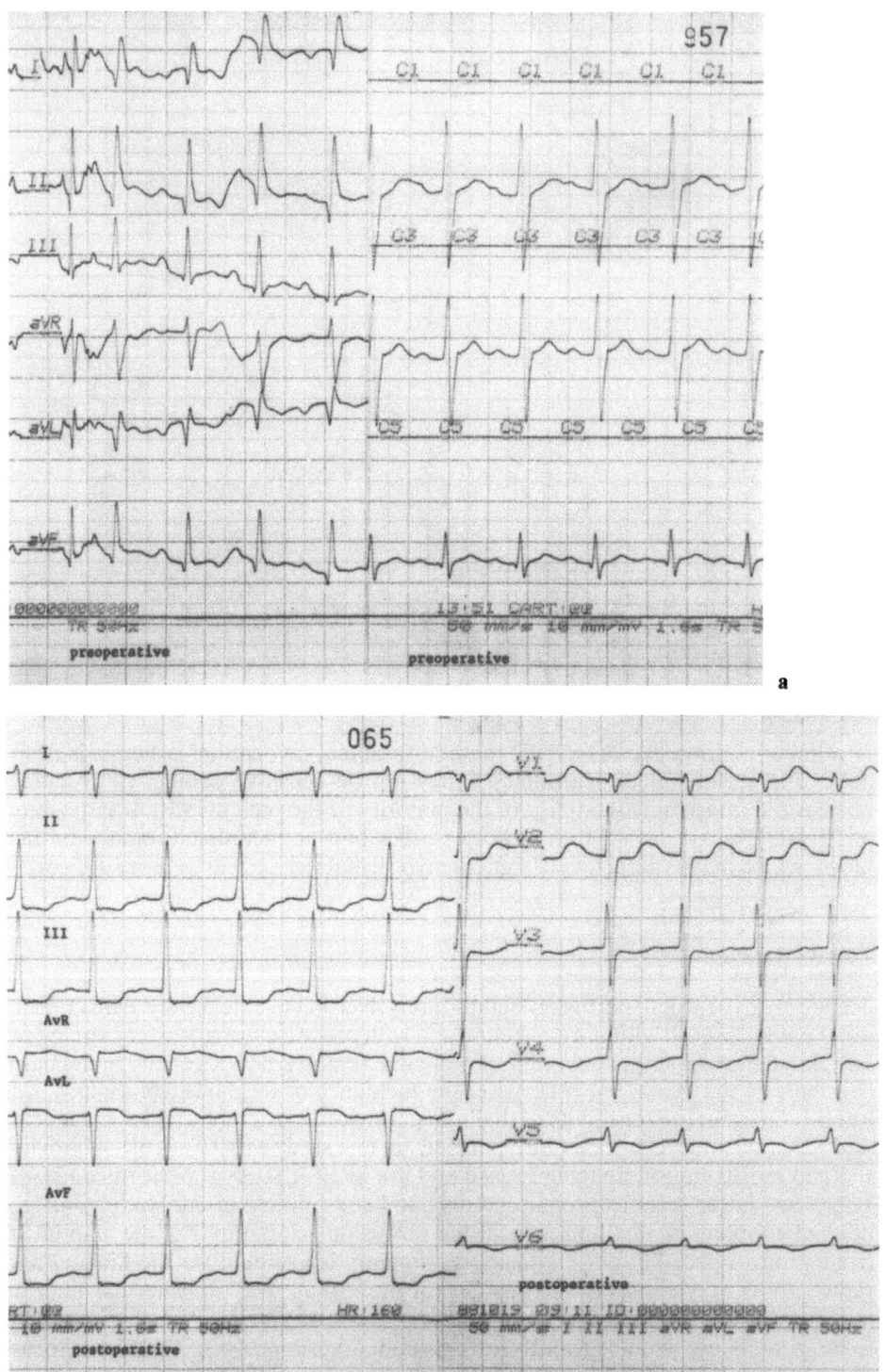

Fig. 3a, b. Pre- (a) and postoperative (b) electrocardiogram in the same patient with wall motion abnormality in the anterolateral left-ventricular wall.

Echocardiography

The main purpose of the preliminary study with thallium perfusion scintigraphy was to define a gold standard to which echocardiographic wall-motion analysis could be compared. Our data suggest that cross-sectional echocardiography in experienced hands provides reproducible evidence of disturbance of regional left-ventricular function which may be due to impairment of myocardial perfusion [19]. Echocardiography is noninvasive, relatively easy to perform, and can be used serially in the evaluation of the patient after an arterial switch operation. Wall-motion analysis is difficult or may be impossible to use in patients who have severe aortic regurgitation [8] or a pacemaker with an abnormal sequence of electrical stimulation and repolarization of the heart [8]. Also, severely impaired global function may limit the accuracy of detection of regional wall-motion abnormalities [13]. The majority of our patients had normal or near normal global left-ventricular function. Only one patient in the Toronto study had a pacemaker and severe aortic regurgitation was absent in all, so that echocardiographic wall-motion analysis could be applied in the vast majority of our patients. If a wall-motion abnormality is detected and has been confirmed by a second observer, we suggest performing a thallium myocardial perfusion scan using either isoproterenol of dypiridamole as pharmacological stress [6]. If the myocardial perfusion scan confirms the finding of impaired myocardial perfusion, we would recommend cardiac catheterization − if possible, with selective angiography in the coronaries, in order to detect or rule out any coronary artery lesions which might be surgically treatable.

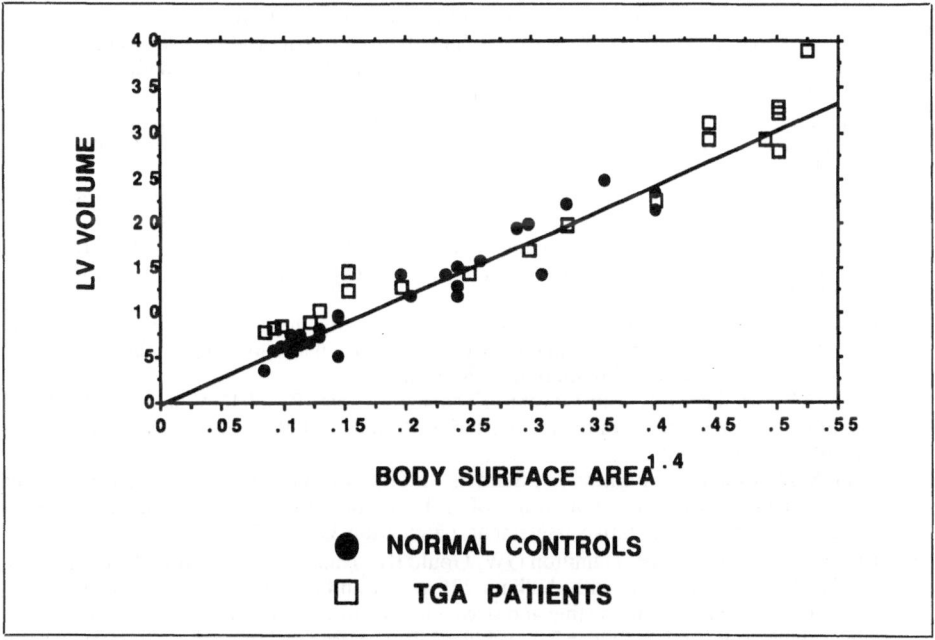

Fig. 4. Left-ventricular volume at last echocardiographic examination in patients with transposition of the great arteries after arterial-switch operation, and in controls with normal hearts.

Conclusions

As a conclusion of both studies, we believe that echocardiographic wall-motion analysis is a sensitive tool to detect myocardial ischemia, if interobserver data are unequivocal. Echocardiographic wall-motion abnormalities due to impairment of myocardial perfusion in newborns with complete transposition of the great arteries are rare after an arterial-switch operation.

References

1. DiDonato RM, Wernovsky G, Walsh EP, Colan SD, Lang P, Wessel DL, Jonas RA, Mayer JE, Castaneda AR (1989) Results of the arterial switch operation for transposition of the great arteries with ventricular septal defect. Circulation 80:1689–1705
2. Garcia EV, van Train K, Maddahi J, Prigent F, Friedman J, Areeda J, Waxman A, Berman DS (1985) Quantification of rotational Thallium-201 myocardial tomography. J Nucl Med 26:17–26
3. Goor DA, Shem-Tov A, Neufeld H (1982) Impeded coronary flow in anatomic correction of transposition of the great arteries. Prevention, detection and managment. J Thorac Cardiovasc Surg 83:747–754
4. Kaul S, Boucher CA, Newell JB, Chesler DA, Greenberg JM, Okada RD, Strauss HW, Dinsmore RE, Pohost GM (1986) Determination of the quantitative thallium imaging variables that optimize detection of coronary artery disease. J Am Coll Cardiol 7:527–537
5. Kirsch CM, Doliwa R, Buell U, Roedler D (1983) Detection of severe coronary heart disease with Tl-201. Comparison of single photon emission tomography with invasive aortography. J Nucl Med 24:761–766
6. Legrand V, Mancini J, Bates ER, Hodgson JM, Gross MD, Vogel RA (1986) Comparative study of coronary flow reserve, coronary anatomy and results of radionuclide exercise test in patients with coronary artery disease. J Am Coll Cardiol 8:1022–1032
7. Lincoln C, Redington AN, Li K, Mattos S, Shinebourne E, Rigby ML (1986) Anatomical correction for complete transposition and double outlet right ventricle: intermediate assessment of functional results. Br Heart J 56:259–266
8. Mann DL, Gillam LD, Weyman AE (1986) Cross sectional echocardiographic assessment of regional left ventricular performance and myocardial perfusion. Progr in Cardiovasc Dis 29:1–52
9. McQueen MJ, Holder D, El-Maraghi NRH (1983) Assessment of accuracy of serial electrocardiograms in the diagnosis of myocardial infarction. Am Heart J 105:258–261
10. Quagebeur JM, Rohmer J, Ottenkamp J, Buis T, Kirklin JW, Blackstone EH, Brom AG (1986) The arterial switch operation: An eight year experience. J Thorac Cardiovasc Surg 92:361–384
11. Parisi AF, Moynihan PF, Folland ED, Feldman CL (1981) Quantitative detection of regional left ventricular contraction abnormalities by two-dimensional echocardiography. II: Accuracy in coronary artery disease. Circulation 63:761–767
12. Planché C, Bruniaux J, Lacour-Gayet F, Kachaner J, Binet JP, Sidi D, Villain E (1988) Switch operation for transposition of the great arteries. A study of 120 patients. J Thorac Cardiovasc Surg 96:354–363
13. Rein AJJT, Colan SD, Parness IA, Sanders SP (1987) Regional and global left ventricular function in infants with anomalous origin of the left coronary artery from the pulmonary trunk: preoperative and postoperative assessment. Circulation 75:115–123
14. Ritchie JL, Trobaugh GB, Hamilton GW, Gould KL, Nahara KA, Murray JA, Williams DL (1977) Myocardial imaging with thallium 201 at rest and during exercise. Comparison with coronary arteriography and resting and stress electrocardiography. Circulation 56:66–73
15. Silverman NH, Ports TA, Snider RA, Schiller NB, Carlsson E, Heilbron DC (1980) Determination of left ventricular volume in children: echocardiographic and angiographic comparisons. Circulation 62:548–557

16. Taylor DN, Choraria SK, Maughan J, Mills J, Pilcher J (1989) Diagnosis of coronary artery disease using thallium imaging: tomographic versus planar imaging. Nucl Med Com 10:401–407
17. Trowitsch E, Colan SD, Sanders SP (1985) Global and regional right ventricular function in normal infants and infants with transposition of the great arteries after Senning operation. Circulation 72:1008–1020
18. Vogel M, Smallhorn JF, Stein JI, Freedom RM (1990) Echocardiographic analysis of regional left ventricular wall motion in normal children and newborns. J Am Coll Cardiol 15:1409–1416
19. Vogel M, Smallhorn JF, Trusler GA, Freedom RM (1990) Echocardiographic analysis of regional left ventricular wall motion in children after the arterial switch operation for complete transposition of the great arteries. J Am Coll Cardiol 15:1417–1423
20. Vogel M, Smallhorn JF, Gilday D, Benson LN, Ash J, Williams WG, Freedom RM (1991) Assessment of myocardial perfusion in patients after the arterial switch. J Nucl Med 32:237–241
21. Vogel M, Staller W, Bühlmeyer K (1991) Left ventricular myocardial mass determined by cross-sectional echocardiography in normal newborns, infants and children. Ped Cardiol 12:143–149
22. Wernovsky G, Hougen TJ, Walsh EP, Sholler GF, Colan SD, Sanders SP, Parness IA, Keane JF, Mayer JE, Jonas RA, Castaneda AR, Lang P (1988) Midterm results after the arterial switch operation for transposition of the great arteries with intact ventricular septum: clinical, hemodynamic, echocardiographic, and electrophysiologic data. Circulation 77:1333–1344

Author's address:
Priv.-Doz. Dr. M. Vogel
Kinderklinik am Deutschen
Herzzentrum München
Lothstr. 11
8000 München 2, FRG

M. Kaltenbach, Frankfurt; R. E. Vlietstra, Lakeland, Florida
Foreword by E. Braunwald, Boston, MA

Concise Cardiology

1991. 180 pp. with 120 figures, 10 tables.
Hardcover DM 60,–
ISBN 3-7985-0864-X (Steinkopff Verlag)
ISBN 0-387-91394-7 (Springer-Verlag New York)

This volume covers the wide range of disciplines in cardiology, and it includes thorough clinical disease-recognition profiles, as well as concise descriptions of therapy methods. Special diagnostic considerations and problems in the management of cardiac and circulatory diseases are discussed, and the information is presented in a logical order. The text has practical significance for both review and for teaching, and the work emphasizes understanding of the material as opposed to just memorization.

Wide acceptance of this work has been demonstrated by the success of the first two German-language editions, authored by Martin Kaltenbach; this first English-language edition represents a cooperation with the American cardiologist R. E. Vlietstra.

Distribution in the USA and Canada through Springer-Verlag, 175 Fifth Avenue, New York, NY 10010; for other countries through your bookseller or directly from Dr. Dietrich Steinkopff Verlag, P. O. Box 11 1442, 6100 Darmstadt/FRG.

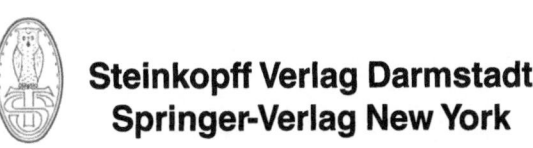
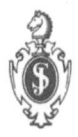

Steinkopff Verlag Darmstadt
Springer-Verlag New York